Women's Health Nurse Practitioner Certification Study Question Book

Beth Kelsey, M.S., R.N.C., N.P.
Women's Health Nurse Practitioner
Instructor
School of Nursing
Ball State University
Muncie, Indiana

Anne Salomone, M.S., R.N.C., C.N.M.
Women's Health Nurse Practitioner
Certified Nurse-Midwife
Stankevych Medical Group
McHenry, Illinois

Clinical Faculty
School of Nursing
Northern Illinois University
Dekalb, Illinois

Health Leadership Associates
Potomac, Maryland

Question Books

Family Nurse Practitioner Certification Study Question Set

(ISBN 1-878028-26-X)

by
Health Leadership Associates, Inc.

Consists of
The

**Adult Nurse Practitioner Certification
Study Question Book
ISBN 1-878028-20-0**

**Pediatric Nurse Practitioner Certification
Study Question Book
ISBN 1-878028-21-9**

**Women's Health Nurse Practitioner
Certification Study Question Book
ISBN 1-878028-22-7**

Additional Nursing Certification Study Question Books by Health Leadership Associates, Inc.

Acute Care Nurse Practitioner Certification Study Question Book
(ISBN# 1-878028-25-1), List Price $30.00

Adult Nurse Practitioner Certification Study Question Book
(ISBN# 1-878028-20-0), List Price $30.00

Pediatric Nurse Practitioner Certification Study Question Book
(ISBN# 1-878028-21-9), List Price $30.00

Women's Health Nurse Practitioner Certification Study Question Book
(ISBN# 1-878028-22-7), List Price $30.00

Family Nurse Practitioner Certification Study Question Book Set
(This shrink wrapped set consists of the Adult, Pediatric, and Women's Health Study Question Books).
(ISBN# 1-878028-26-X). List Price $60.00

Health Leadership Associates, Inc.
Managing Editor: Virginia Layng Millonig
                Mary A. Millonig
Manuscript Editor: Sally K. Miller
Production Manager: Martha M. Pounsberry
Editorial Assistants: Bridget M. Jones
                Cheryl C. Patterson
Cover and Design: Merrifield Graphics
Composition: Port City Press, Inc.
Design and Production: Port City Press, Inc.

Copyright © 1999 by Health Leadership Associates, Inc.

Printed in the United States of America

Health Leadership Associates, Inc.
P.O. Box 59153
Potomac, Maryland 20859

Library of Congress Cataloging-in-Publication Data

Kelsey, Beth.
  Women's health nurse practitioner certification study question
book / Beth Kelsey, Anne Salomone.
      p. cm. — (Family nurse practitioner certification study
question set)
  Includes bibliographical references.
  ISBN 1-878028-22-7 (paperback)
  1. Gynecologic nursing—Examinations Study guides.   2. Nurse
Practitioners—Examinations Study guides.   I. Salomone, Anne.
II. Title.   III. Series.
  [DNLM: 1. Genital Diseases, Female—nursing Examination Questions.
2. Nurse Practitioners Examination Questions.   3. Nursing Care
Examination Questions.   4. Obstetrical Nursing Examination
Questions.   5. Women's Health Examination Questions.   WY 18.2 K29w
1999]
RG105.K45   1999
610.73'678'076—dc21
DNLM/DLC
for Library of Congress   99-22640
                                                    CIP

10 9 8 7 6 5 4
Fourth printing June 2003

Reviewers

Preface

Health Leadership Associates is pleased to introduce one more component to our complement of Nurse Practitioner Certification Review materials. This ''Women's Health Nurse Practitioner Certification Study Question Book'' will further assist the user of this book to be successful in the examination process. It should by no means be the only source used for preparation for the Women's Health Nurse Practitioner Certification examination nor the Family Nurse Practitioner Certification examination. It has been developed primarily to enhance your test taking skills while also integrating the principles (becoming test-wise) of test taking found in the ''Test Taking Strategies and Skills'' chapter of both the ''Women's Health Care Nurse Practitioner Certification Review Guide''and the ''Adult Nurse Practitioner Certification Review Guide'' published by Health Leadership Associates. These review guides, in addition to the review courses and home study programs, provide a comprehensive and total approach to success in the examination process. It enables the users of these materials to be successful in the test taking process, and reinforces the knowledge base that is critical in the delivery of care in the practice setting. Many individuals feel that taking practice test questions is the most important factor in the certification examination preparation process, yet it is but one strategy to be used in combination with a strong knowledge base. Success in the certification examination area is based upon both excellent test taking skills and a comprehensive understanding of the content of the examination. As a nurse practitioner seeking certification, it is important to not lose sight of the definition and purpose of certification. ''Certification is an evaluative process that provides nurses or nurse practitioners in the obstetric, gynecologic and/or neonatal nursing specialty the opportunity to publicly demonstrate what they know and to be recognized for the knowledge they possess (National Certification Corporation for the Obstetric, Gynecologic and Neonatal Nursing Specialties, 1997). According to the American Nurses Association, ''Certification is a process by which nongovernmental agencies or associations confirm that an individual licensed to practice as a professional has met certain predetermined standards specified by that profession for specialty practice. Its purpose is to assure the public that an individual has mastered a body of knowledge and acquired skills in a particular specialty'' (American Nurses Association, 1979).

Inherent to the preparation for certification examinations is rigorous attention to the directives and materials from the certification boards. Content outlines and sample test questions are often provided to examinees prior to the examinations. Specifics for each examination including suggested readings will be provided by the individual testing boards.

This question book has been prepared by board certified nurse practitioners. The questions have then been reviewed and critiqued by board certified nurse practitioners (content experts) and a test construction specialist. There are 300 problem oriented certification board-type multiple choice questions which are divided according to content area (based upon testing board content outlines) with answers, rationales and a reference list. Every effort has been made to develop sample questions that are representative of the types of questions that may be found on the certification examinations, however, style and format of the examination may differ. Engaging in the exercise of test taking, an understanding of test taking strategies, and knowledge in respective content areas can only lead to success.

CONTENTS

Primary Care

Beth Kelsey
Anne Salomone

Select one best answer to the following questions.

Questions 1 and 2 refer to the following scenario.

A 66-year-old woman presents to your office for her annual examination in November. She had a mammogram, Pap smear, and test for fecal occult blood one year ago. She had a screening sigmoidoscopy two years ago. She had her last tetanus-diphtheria (Td) 12 years ago. She had her pneumococcal and influenza vaccinations one year ago.

1. Which of the following screening tests should be performed or ordered at this visit?

    a. Mammogram and Pap smear
    b. Mammogram, Pap smear, and fecal occult blood
    c. Mammogram, Pap smear, and sigmoidoscopy
    d. Pap smear and fecal occult blood

2. What vaccinations would be recommended at the current visit?

    a. Influenza only
    b. Influenza and pneumococcal
    c. Influenza and Td booster
    d. Influenza, pneumococcal, and Td booster

Questions 3 and 4 refer to the following scenario.

A 40-year-old woman has no family history of heart disease. Her weight and blood pressure are within normal limits and she does not smoke.

3. Which of the following laboratory results for this woman would indicate the need for a lipoprotein analysis to include LDL?

    a. Cholesterol 225 mg/dL, HDL 65 mg/dL
    b. Cholesterol 220 mg/dL, HDL 25 mg/dL
    c. Cholesterol 215 mg/dL, HDL 45 mg/dL
    d. Cholesterol 200 mg/dL, HDL 55 mg/dL

4. What dietary recommendations for prevention of heart disease should be included when counseling this woman?

    a. Limit fat intake to no more than 30% of daily calories
    b. Foods that are low in cholesterol will also be low in fat
    c. Foods from plant sources do not contain any saturated fat
    d. No more than 50% of daily calories should be saturated fat

Questions 5 and 6 refer to the following scenario.

A 30-year-old woman presents to your office requesting assistance with efforts to quit smoking. She currently smokes one pack per day.

5. She is concerned about gaining weight if she quits smoking. The appropriate response would be to tell her that:

    a. The majority of smokers do not gain any weight when they quit smoking
    b. A smoker should expect to gain 15 to 20 pounds the first year after quitting
    c. The average weight gain during smoking cessation is about 7 to 10 pounds
    d. Weight gained during smoking cessation is easily lost in a few months

6. She decides she would like to use nicotine replacement patches to help her quit smoking. Instructions concerning the use of nicotine replacement patches include telling her to:

    a. Begin to taper the number of cigarettes smoked when she starts the patches
    b. Discontinue smoking for at least one week before starting the patches
    c. Start to use the patches on the first day that she does not smoke
    d. Wait one week after starting the patches to discontinue smoking

7. A 22-year-old woman presents to your office with a history suggestive of irritable bowel syndrome. Which of the following symptoms would you expect to be present?

    a. Frequent awakening at night with abdominal cramps
    b. Weight loss related to nausea and loss of appetite
    c. Increase in severity of symptoms with physical activity
    d. Abdominal pain or discomfort relieved with defecation

8. Which of the following pharmacologic treatments for constipation would be most appropriate for a patient with irritable bowel syndrome?

    a. Bulk forming agents
    b. Osmotic laxatives
    c. Stimulant laxatives
    d. Stool softeners

9. A 26-year-old woman presents with abrupt onset diarrhea that started 24 hours ago. She has had approximately six loose stools without any noticeable blood. She has mild abdominal cramping, no nausea, and no fever. Initial management of this patient should include:

    a. Advising liquids rich in electrolytes and sugar
    b. Advising high protein liquid supplements
    c. Obtaining a stool sample for culture
    d. Initiating treatment with antimicrobials

10. A 32-year-old woman presents with a three month history of intermittent burning retrosternal pain that radiates to her back. Symptoms are noted 30 to 60 minutes after eating and are relieved quickly by the use of antacids. There is no relationship of symptoms to exercise or exertion. Physical examination and vital signs are within normal limits (WNL). The most likely diagnosis is:

    a. Acute cholecystitis
    b. Gastric ulcer disease
    c. Gastroesophageal reflux
    d. Ischemic heart disease

11. A 26-year-old obese woman presents with colicky right upper quadrant pain radiating to the mid-upper back. She also complains of nausea and vomiting. Oral temperature is 100.2° F. She has a positive Murphy's sign upon direct palpation of the right upper quadrant. Considering the history and examination findings, the principle diagnostic test to order is a/an:

    a. Abdominal ultrasound
    b. Endoscopy with biopsy
    c. Stool culture and sensitivity
    d. Upper GI barium radiograph

Questions 12 and 13 refer to the following scenario.

A 14-year-old sexually active female presents to your office for contraception. She has been having heavy periods since menarche six months ago and now has a hemoglobin of 11.5 g/dL. Her physical examination is normal. She is started on oral contraceptives and ferrous sulfate.

12. One week after starting her iron therapy, the patient calls to tell you that the iron pills make her sick to her stomach and give her heartburn. An appropriate action would be to:

    a. Advise her to take her iron with an antacid
    b. Advise her to take her iron with orange juice
    c. Suggest that she take her iron pills with meals
    d. Switch from oral iron therapy to IM injections

13. Three months later her Hgb is 14 g/dL and her periods are regulated. An appropriate test to determine if her iron stores have been replenished is a:

    a. Total iron binding capacity
    b. Plasma transferrin level
    c. Reticulocyte count
    d. Serum ferritin level

14. An African-American couple planning a pregnancy presents to your office with questions about sickle cell anemia. Both of them carry the sickle cell trait. She has a brother who has sickle cell disease. The likelihood that their child will have sickle cell disease is:

    a. 0%
    b. 25%
    c. 50%
    d. 100%

15. The definitive test for sickle cell anemia is the:

    a. Hgb electrophoresis
    b. Indirect Coombs

c. Sickledex preparation
d. Schilling test

Questions 16, 17, and 18 refer to the following scenario.

When taking a health history on a 35-year-old woman, you learn that she has a history of migraine headaches. She tells you that in the last year they have occurred two to three times each month. She takes over-the-counter pain medication and has to go to bed when she has the headaches.

16. Which of the following characteristics is not typically associated with migraine headaches?
    a. The headache is often accompanied by nausea
    b. The age of onset is usually > 30
    c. The headaches can last for up to 72 hours
    d. The location of the pain is usually unilateral

17. Because this patient's headaches are occurring two or more times each month, preventive therapy is being considered. Which of the following medications is indicated for preventive therapy of migraine headaches?
    a. Beta-adrenergic blocking agents
    b. Codeine containing analgesics
    c. Ergotamine preparations
    d. Sumatriptan

18. If sumatriptan is prescribed, the client should be instructed that:
    a. This medication should be taken at the onset of a headache before taking any other pain medications
    b. The effectiveness of this medication can be improved when combined with an ergotamine
    c. A common side effect of this medication is nausea and vomiting
    d. This medication should be used with caution due to its addictive potential

Questions 19 and 20 refer to the following scenario.

A 30-year-old female who does repetitive small parts work in a factory presents with the complaint of intermittent numbness and tingling in the fingers of her right hand.

19. Physical examination reveals a positive Tinel's sign and a positive Phalen's maneuver. These two tests are usually positive with:

    a. Multiple sclerosis
    b. Raynaud's phenomenon
    c. Carpal tunnel syndrome
    d. Stress fractures of the wrist

20. Considering the patient's symptoms and the two positive tests, what other findings would you expect?

    a. Blanching of the fingers when cold
    b. Excess sweating of the hand palms
    c. Neck pain that radiates down the arm
    d. Increase in symptoms during the night

21. A 28-year-old obese female who recently started working in housekeeping at the hospital presents in your office with low back pain. If her back pain is caused by lumbosacral muscle strain, expected symptoms and examination findings would include:

    a. Diminished knee jerk reflexes
    b. Increased pain with forward bending
    c. Positive straight leg raise test
    d. Radiation of pain down one leg

22. The patient with low back pain related to lumbosacral strain should be advised that:

    a. Abdominal strengthening exercises help to prevent recurrence
    b. Heat therapy, rather than cold packs, should be used for pain relief
    c. One to two weeks of bedrest may be necessary for full recovery
    d. Back stretching exercises are an important part of therapy

23. Which of the following history or physical examination findings is characteristic of osteoarthritis?

    a. Crepitus upon movement of the affected joints
    b. Joint pain that gets worse as the day progresses
    c. Soft tissue swelling around the affected joints
    d. Presence of fatigue and general malaise

24. A 34-year-old female presents with complaints of fatigue and generalized muscle and joint pain for the past several months. She has normal range of motion,

no apparent swelling of joints, and no abnormal neurological findings. She has multiple tender points over the muscles on both sides of her body when pressure is applied. Sites of tenderness include the suboccipital, trapezius, and gluteal muscles. A probable diagnosis is:

a. Fibromyalgia
b. Lupus erythematosus
c. Polymyalgia rheumatica
d. Rheumatoid arthritis

Questions 25 and 26 refer to the following scenario.

25. A 32-year-old female presents with a recent onset of irregular patches of erythema and oozing vesicles on her hands. She complains of itching and burning of the affected areas. The most likely cause is:

a. Contact dermatitis
b. Fungal infection
c. Cellulitis
d. Scabies

26. Appropriate treatment for this condition is:

a. Erythromycin
b. Ketoconazole
c. Permethrin 5% cream
d. Topical corticosteroids

27. A 25-year-old female presents in your office for her annual examination. You notice a 5 cm annular lesion with a pale center on her leg. She states it does not itch and that she first noticed it about one week after returning from a camping trip she took last month. A likely diagnosis is:

a. Cellulitis
b. Lyme disease
c. Poison ivy
d. Spider bite

28. A 56-year-old female presents with a mole on the back of her neck that started bleeding when she was drying the area with a towel. She was unaware that she had this mole prior to its bleeding. In examining the area the nurse practitioner should keep in mind that:

a. The most common form of skin cancer is malignant melanoma
b. The characteristic lesion seen with melanoma has a rolled border
c. Malignant melanoma is uncommon in this age group
d. The diameter of a melanoma is usually greater than 6 mm

29. A 50-year-old African-American female tells you her father had glaucoma, and asks if there is a test she can get to see if she could have glaucoma. You could appropriately advise this patient that:

    a. Screening for glaucoma is recommended every three years after age 65
    b. Screening for glaucoma should be done yearly using a Schiötz tonometer
    c. She should see an ophthalmologist for regular glaucoma screening
    d. Glaucoma screening is only needed if she is having vision changes

30. A 22-year-old female presents with the complaint that for the past 24 hours her right eye has felt "scratchy" and had a watery discharge. She reports no problems with vision and no photophobia. Examination reveals peripheral injection with watery discharge in the right eye. A likely cause for her symptoms is:

    a. Allergic conjunctivitis
    b. Corneal abrasion
    c. Subconjunctival hemorrhage
    d. Viral conjunctivitis

Questions 31 and 32 refer to the following scenario.

A 27-year-old woman confides in you that her husband has been both emotionally and physically abusive to her over the past several years. She says that since the last abuse two weeks ago he has actually been very attentive and has promised to quit drinking.

31. An appropriate initial plan of care for this woman would include encouragement to:

    a. Discuss the abuse that has occurred in specific and concrete terms
    b. Discuss what she has done differently in the past two weeks
    c. Leave the situation immediately and seek legal recourse
    d. Talk with her partner about seeing a counselor as a couple

32. In relation to the cycle of violence, you could describe to the woman how her husband's current behavior is typical of the:

    a. Tension building phase

b. Recovery phase
c. Honeymoon phase
d. Reality phase

33. A 30-year-old woman comes to your office for follow-up of minor injuries sustained in a car accident. She admits that she was arrested for driving under the influence of alcohol, and that her husband has moved out because of her drinking. She states that she did quit drinking for a few days after the accident, but felt like she was going to crawl out of her skin. Which of the following pieces of information would suggest that she has an alcohol dependency?

    a. She drinks in situations in which alcohol use is physically hazardous
    b. She has interpersonal problems related to her alcohol use
    c. She has repeated legal problems directly related to alcohol use
    d. She makes unsuccessful attempts to cut down or control alcohol use

34. Which of the following would be considered a risk factor for both type 2 diabetes and coronary heart disease in a 45-year-old woman?

    a. Waist to hip ratio of 0.7
    b. Central body fat distribution
    c. 20% above desirable weight
    d. Body mass index of 25

35. A 40-year-old woman who is 20 pounds overweight wants to start a weight loss regimen. She smokes ½ pack daily but has no other major risk factors for cardiovascular disease. It would be appropriate to advise this patient that:

    a. Aerobic exercise may help to increase her basal metabolic rate
    b. Aerobic exercise may cause a problem with increase in appetite
    c. Prior to starting any exercise she needs an exercise tolerance test
    d. She should quit smoking prior to initiating an exercise program

36. Similarities between the two eating disorders of anorexia nervosa and bulimia include:

    a. Substance abuse as an accompanying problem
    b. Amenorrhea as part of the diagnostic criteria
    c. Lack of control as a predominating feature
    d. Depression often accompanies the eating disorder

Questions 37 and 38 refer to the following scenario.

A 35-year-old female has been diagnosed with major depression. She states that she has had several symptoms of depression for the past month including loss of appetite, insomnia, loss of energy, and inability to concentrate.

37. To meet the DSM-IV diagnostic criteria for major depression she must also exhibit:

   a. Feelings of worthlessness or excessive guilt
   b. Thoughts about dying or committing suicide
   c. Loss of interest or pleasure in most activities
   d. Previous occurrence of the same symptoms

38. Her physician has prescribed trazodone (a heterocyclic antidepressant), and paroxetine (a serotonin reuptake inhibitor), as part of her treatment. Client education should include instructing her that:

   a. They should be taken on alternating days to avoid an overdose
   b. They should both be taken at night for optimal effect
   c. She should try both separately and decide which is most helpful
   d. Paroxetine should be taken in the morning and trazodone at night

39. In relation to the current leading cause of death in children and adolescents, one of the most important topics for anticipatory guidance for a 16-year-old female would include discussion about:

   a. Always wearing seat belts in the car
   b. Annual Pap smears if she is sexually active
   c. Monthly self breast examination
   d. Condom use and abstinence

40. A 24-year-old normal weight, nonpregnant female gives the following 24 hour diet recall: Breakfast — 1 serving of cereal, 1 banana, 1 glass milk, 1 cup coffee; lunch — cheeseburger on bun, baked potato, coke; snack — 1 apple; dinner — 2 servings chicken, 1 serving broccoli, salad, 1 glass milk; snack — 1 cup of yogurt. According to the Food Guide Pyramid recommendations she is low in:

   a. Milk group
   b. Vegetable group
   c. Fruit group
   d. Bread group

41. Routine health screening aimed at early detection of the leading causes of death in women 50 to 64 years of age includes:

    a. Cholesterol, HDL (annually), sigmoidoscopy (every 3 to 5 years), and Pap smear (every 1 to 3 years)
    b. Cholesterol, HDL (every 3 to 5 years), Pap smear (every 1 to 3 years), and mammography (annually)
    c. Mammography (annually), cholesterol, HDL (every 5 years) and fecal occult blood testing (annually)
    d. Pap smear (every 1 to 3 years), fecal occult blood testing (annually), and sigmoidoscopy (every 3 to 5 years)

42. A 50-year-old premenopausal woman presents for her routine annual examination. Her blood pressure is 145/90 mm Hg. Her weight is within normal limits, she is a nonsmoker, and drinks a glass of wine with dinner each night. She does not engage in any regular exercise. Her family history includes both her father and grandfather having myocardial infarctions when they were in their late 50s. Management for this client should include:

    a. Decreasing alcohol intake to no more than 2 to 3 glasses of wine each week
    b. Monitoring blood pressure every six months as it is currently borderline
    c. Encouraging aerobic physical activity 30 to 45 minutes most days of the week
    d. Starting estrogen replacement therapy to decrease risk for myocardial infarction

43. A 45-year-old female has a cardiovascular profile drawn. The results include a total cholesterol 240 mg/dL, HDL 50 mg/dL, LDL 115 mg/dL and cholesterol/HDL ratio of 4.5. Which of these laboratory values would warrant further evaluation?

    a. Total cholesterol
    b. HDL value
    c. LDL value
    d. Cholesterol/HDL ratio

44. The menopausal female most at risk for coronary artery disease would be one who is:

    a. 5'4" tall, weighs 125 lbs, is on estrogen replacement therapy, and smokes $\frac{1}{2}$ pack daily

    b. 5'5" tall, weighs 140 lbs, is not on estrogen replacement therapy, and doesn't smoke

    c. 5'6" tall, weighs 145 lbs, is on estrogen replacement therapy, and smokes $\frac{1}{2}$ pack daily

    d. 5'7" tall, weighs 185 lbs, is not on estrogen replacement therapy, and smokes $\frac{1}{2}$ pack daily

45. A 22-year-old female presents with complaints of intermittent palpitations and occasional chest pain that she describes as sharp and not related to exertion. She is 5'2", 106 lbs., and has normal vital signs. She does not smoke and is not on any medication. Her physical examination is normal except for a mid-systolic click and a systolic murmur. The most useful test to confirm her likely diagnosis would be a/an:

    a. Chest radiograph
    b. Cardiac enzyme panel
    c. Echocardiogram
    d. Electrocardiogram

46. Which of the following physical examination findings would correlate with an elevated TSH and a suppressed FT_4 level?

    a. Exophthalmos
    b. Nystagmus
    c. Periorbital edema
    d. Ptosis of the eyelids

47. The usual sequence of female pubertal events is:

    a. Breast development, growth of pubic and axillary hair, menses, peak increase in height
    b. Breast development, growth of pubic and axillary hair, peak increase in height, menses
    c. Peak increase in height, breast development, menses, growth of pubic and axillary hair
    d. Growth of pubic and axillary hair, peak increase in height, breast development, menses

48. A 24-year-old female presents with a mild sore throat for the past two weeks and a temperature of 99.8° F. She also complains of anorexia and feeling ''run down.'' She thinks this may be due to the stress of her recent final exams at school, and a recent break up with her boyfriend. Physical examination findings include pharyngeal exudate, petechiae on her soft palate, and cervical

lymphadenopathy. Considering her age, history, symptoms, and examination findings, which of the following tests would most likely be positive?

 a. Gonorrhea culture from the throat
 b. Heterophil antibody blood test
 c. Rapid strep antibody screen
 d. Tzanck smear from soft palate

49. Which of the following is not considered to be a risk factor for the development of type 2 diabetes?

 a. Alcohol abuse
 b. Hispanic race
 c. Hyperlipidemia
 d. Hypertension

50. A 35-year-old female presents with a complaint of nervousness, increased perspiration, weight loss despite an increased appetite, and frequent bowel movements. Abnormal examination findings include patellar reflexes 3+, heart rate 100 bpm, and a moderately enlarged, soft, nontender thyroid gland. The most likely diagnosis is:

 a. Graves' disease
 b. Hypothyroidism
 c. Myxedema
 d. Thyroiditis

51. A 32-year-old female with asthma presents for her annual examination. She relates that she has been taking propranolol for three months for migraine prophylaxis. She has continued with her usual asthma medications of an albuterol inhaler and theophylline. She states she has had a nonproductive cough and has had to use her inhaler more frequently. Her physical examination is within normal limits except for an expiratory wheeze. Appropriate actions would include:

 a. Advising her to see her physician for evaluation of her medications
 b. Administering a PPD skin test and ordering a chest radiograph
 c. Encouraging fluids and having her return for evaluation in one week
 d. Obtaining a throat culture and initiating antibiotic therapy

52. A 60-year-old female presents with pleuritic chest pain and a cough productive of yellow sputum. Her temperature is 101.0° F, respiratory rate is 32 bpm, and her heart rate is 90 bpm. She appears to be somewhat dehydrated. Expected findings on physical examination would include:

  a. Decreased vocal fremitus
  b. Jugular venous distention
  c. Areas of dullness over lungs
  d. Absence of bronchophony

53. A 19-year-old female, who is a steroid dependent asthmatic, presents to your office for her physical examination for college. Her immunizations are up to date and she had a negative Tine test six months ago. Her only medications are oral contraceptives and asthma medications including daily prednisone. The physical examination form that she presents requires demonstration of testing for TB within the past 12 months. Given the above history you advise her that:

  a. The Tine test should be repeated in one year
  b. A Mantoux test should be administered in six months
  c. A PPD skin test for TB may be unreliable
  d. A PPD skin test is contraindicated due to her asthma

54. According to the CDC criteria for preventive therapy of tuberculosis, an individual with a PPD test showing an induration of ≥ 5 mm should receive treatment if she:

  a. Currently lives in a long term care facility
  b. Has had contact with an active TB case
  c. Is over 35 years old regardless of risk factors
  d. Previously received a BCG vaccination

55. A 67-year-old Hispanic female, who lives with her son and his seven children in a tenement building, presents with respirations of 32 bpm and a temperature of 101° F. She was hospitalized a year ago for a stroke and has had difficulty eating. She is not able to tell you how long she has been sick or how she got to the clinic today. You make the diagnosis of pneumonia. Her risk factors for a complicated course include:

  a. Hispanic race, living with children, temperature of 101° F
  b. Mental confusion, age over 65, temperature of 101° F
  c. Living with children, living in a tenement building, temperature of 101° F
  d. Living in a tenement building, Hispanic race, temperature of 101° F

56. A client comes to your office for a routine examination and needs an MMR vaccine and TB test. Appropriate timing for the vaccination and TB test would be to:

  a. Delay the TB testing for six weeks from the time of the MMR

    b. Give only the rubella vaccine and the TB test at this visit

    c. Delay the rubella vaccine for four weeks after the TB test is given

    d. Give the MMR and have the client return in two weeks for the TB test

57. Which of the following is diagnostic of HIV?

    a. Positive ELISA, negative Western blot

    b. Negative ELISA, positive Western blot

    c. Negative ELISA, negative Western blot

    d. Positive ELISA, positive Western blot

58. Which of the following would provide the best measure of long term control of diabetes?

    a. Three hour glucose tolerance test

    b. Absence of vascular complications

    c. Daily blood glucose levels

    d. Hemoglobin A_{1c}

59. A 33-year-old female recently saw a show on chronic fatigue syndrome. She tells you that she thinks she may have this condition because she has been extremely fatigued for the past month and has had pain in her joints. In evaluating this client you will want to take into consideration that:

    a. A diagnosis of chronic fatigue syndrome requires that symptoms persist for at least three months

    b. Symptoms commonly include sore throat, headaches, and both joint and muscle pain

    c. This condition occurs most frequently during the perimenopause and is likely hormone related

    d. Physical findings commonly include joint inflammation, muscle weakness, and generalized lymphadenopathy

60. Treatment for chronic fatigue syndrome includes:

    a. Advice to avoid multivitamin supplementation

    b. Discussing the potential benefits of counseling

    c. Initiation of low doses of fluoxetine

    d. Initiation of a rigorous aerobic exercise routine

Answers and Rationale

1. **(b)** The American Cancer Society (ACS) and American College of Obstetricians and Gynecologists (ACOG) have the following cancer screening recommendations: Women age 50 and older should have annual mammograms (ACS now recommends that annual mammograms start at age 40), Pap smear every 1 to 3 years starting at onset of sexual activity or at 18 years of age, fecal occult blood testing annually starting at age 50, and sigmoidoscopy every 3 to 5 years (ACOG) every 5 years (ACS) starting at age 50 (DHHS, pp. 247, 259, 265, 298).

2. **(c)** Major authorities, including the American Academy of Family Physicians and the U.S. Preventive Services Task Force (USPSTF) have the following immunization recommendations: Influenza immunization should be given annually to all individuals 65 or older, all immunocompetent individuals age 65 and older should be immunized once with pneumococcal vaccine, and adults should receive a tetanus-diphtheria (Td) booster vaccination every 10 years (DHHS, pp. 345, 354, 365).

3. **(b)** The National Cholesterol Education Program (NCEP) of the National Heart, Lung and Blood Institute recommends that lipoprotein analysis be performed in *any* of the following situations: HDL less than 35 mg/dL, total cholesterol 240 mg/dL or greater, a cholesterol of 200-239 mg/dL in an individual with two or more coronary heart disease (CHD) risk factors, or if an individual has CHD. HDL has a protective effect against CHD (DHHS, p. 223).

4. **(a)** The American Heart Association (AHA) recommends that no more than 30% of daily calories should come from fat. Saturated fat should not exceed 10% of total fat intake. All dietary cholesterol comes from animal products. Some saturated fats come from both animal and plant sources. A food can be high in saturated fat but contain no cholesterol. An example is peanut butter (Millonig, p. 120).

5. **(c)** The average weight gain during smoking cessation is about 7 to 10 lbs. The client who is attempting smoking cessation may also need assistance planning diet and exercise routines. The problem of weight gain during smoking cessation is important to address. It is one of the most frequently

cited concerns of women smokers. It is also one of the major causes of relapse (Star, et al., pp. 14-59).

6. **(c)** Nicotine replacement patch use is contraindicated while the client is still smoking. Because withdrawal symptoms may begin shortly after smoking is discontinued, use of the patches should be initiated as soon as the client stops smoking. Although the client may start use of the patches several days after she quits smoking, this is not necessary (DHHS, p. 437).

7. **(d)** Criteria for the diagnosis of irritable bowel syndrome includes continuous or recurrent symptoms, for at least three months, of abdominal pain or discomfort relieved with defecation or associated with a change in frequency or consistency of stool. The individual must also have an irregular pattern of defecation at least 25% of the time with three or more of the following: Altered stool frequency, altered stool form, altered stool passage, passage of mucus and bloating, or feeling of abdominal distention. Typically IBS does not awaken the individual nor does it result in significant weight loss. Physical activity generally does not cause an increase in severity of symptoms and regular physical exercise may benefit the individual with IBS (Carlson, et al., pp. 79-80; Dains, et al., p. 192).

8. **(a)** Increasing dietary fiber will result in a bulkier stool and is considered appropriate treatment for both diarrhea and constipation in IBS. Bulk forming agents such as psyllium husk fiber and methylcellulose can also be used for this purpose (Carlson, et al., p. 81; Lommel & Jackson, p. 325).

9. **(a)** Acute diarrhea is usually self-limiting. Food should be restricted, but oral hydration should be maintained with fluids rich in electrolytes. Restart foods slowly as tolerated with clear liquids and then carbohydrates. Resume protein and fats last. Stool culture may be indicated if symptoms persist and/or if the client has fever or bloody stools (Blackwell, p. 178).

10. **(c)** The intermittent nature, location, and timing of the pain, along with its association of relief with antacids, is highly suggestive of gastroesophageal reflux disease (GERD). If there is suspicion of heart disease, or other disorders, appropriate evaluation is indicated (Star, et al., pp. 7-37).

11. **(a)** History and physical examination are indicative of cholecystitis. Abdominal

ultrasound is the principle diagnostic test for cholelithiasis which is the most common cause of cholecystitis (Blackwell, p. 184).

12. **(c)** Approximately 15% to 20% of individuals experience gastrointestinal side effects with oral iron supplementation. While iron is better absorbed on an empty stomach, ingesting it with food may decrease gastric irritation so that the individual will continue to take the iron. Other options would be to try a different iron preparation or to slowly increase dosage. While vitamin C increases absorption, taking her iron with orange juice will probably not alleviate gastric irritation. Antacids inhibit absorption. IM iron injections are usually not required (Carr, et al., pp. 623-624).

13. **(d)** Serum ferritin is the major iron storage protein. It is present in serum concentrations directly related to iron stores (Richer, p. 95).

14. **(b)** If both parents are carriers of the sickle cell trait, they each have one affected gene and one normal gene for the disorder. Each offspring has a 25% chance of receiving the affected gene from both parents. In an autosomal recessive disorder both genes must be affected for the individual to have the disease (Lowdermilk, et al., p. 109).

15. **(a)** Hgb electrophoresis is the test of choice for distinguishing between the carrier and the affected state. It is very accurate in identifying the types of hemoglobin in a blood sample. Sickledex preparation is a commonly used screening test. A positive Sickledex must be confirmed with Hgb electrophoresis (DHHS, p. 186)

16. **(b)** Migraine headaches usually begin in adolescence or early adulthood. Migraine headaches are typically unilateral, can last up to 72 hours, and are often accompanied by nausea (Carr, et al., pp. 610-611).

17. **(a)** Beta-adrenergic blocking agents such as propranolol are indicated for preventive therapy of migraine headache. The other three medications are indicated for abortive therapy of acute migraine headaches (Carr, et al., pp. 613-614).

18. **(a)** Sumatriptan should be taken at the onset of a headache for best results. It has the beneficial effect of also helping to relieve nausea. It should not be

used if ergotamine preparations have been used in the past 24 hours. Suma-triptan is not considered to carry a risk for addiction (Star, et al., pp. 9-26; Carr, et al., p. 612).

19. **(c)** Carpel tunnel syndrome is caused by compression or irritation of the me-dian nerve at the wrist. Often there is no apparent predisposing cause, but overuse activities with repetitive flexion at the wrist or pincer motion may precipitate this syndrome. Typical symptoms include a dull aching pain across the wrist and forearm with paresthesia, weakness, or clumsiness of the hand. Tinel's sign is elicited by tapping over the median nerve at the palmar surface of the wrist. Tinel's sign is positive when the client has a tingling or prickling sensation along the first 3 digits, wrist pain and weak grip. Phalen's sign is positive when the client experiences numbness and paraesthesia in the fingers innervated by the median nerve after maintaining palmar flexion for one minute. These are both seen with carpal tunnel syn-drome (Dains, et al., pp. 345-346).

20. **(d)** Nocturnal pain and radiation of pain up to the proximal forearm are also common symptomatology with Carpal tunnel syndrome. Examination find-ings, in addition to positive Tinel's and Phalen's signs may include muscle atrophy and dry skin on the affected hand (Dains, et al., pp. 345-346).

21. **(b)** Symptoms of lumbosacral muscle strain include pain in the back and but-tocks, frequently following new activity. The pain is increased with range of motion of the spine, especially flexion. Examination findings would not include any abnormal neurological findings. If pain is elicited with straight leg raises, consider nerve root involvement such as sciatica (Dains, et al., p. 363).

22. **(a)** Abdominal strengthening exercises are useful in preventing recurrence of back strain. The use of heat, cold packs, or the combination of both can be useful in providing relief of back pain. Bedrest is not recommended as part of therapy for lumbosacral strain. Back stretching exercises have been shown to be of little value and are not recommended (Jones, p. 68).

23. **(a)** Osteoarthritis is a degenerative disease of the cartilage of joints. It is the most common form of chronic arthritis affecting up to $\frac{1}{4}$ of the adult popu-lation. Common presenting history is asymmetrical joint pain and stiffness

that improves throughout the day. Joints involved typically include the distal and proximal interphalangeal joints, hips, knees, and the cervical and lumbar spine. Physical examination findings typically include crepitus and limited range of motion of the joints. The joints feel cool with bony enlargement. Constitutional signs such as fatigue and malaise are not characteristic of osteoarthritis (Ross, pp. 23-24).

24. **(a)** Fibromyalgia is characterized by unexplained widespread pain or aching, persistent fatigue, generalized morning stiffness, nonrefreshing sleep and multiple tender points. Pain over specific point sites can be elicited with digital pressure over these areas. Findings are bilateral and involve both the upper and lower body. Changes in range of motion, swelling in the joints, and abnormal neurological findings are not characteristic of fibromyalgia (Maurizio & Rogers, pp. 19-20).

25. **(a)** Contact dermatitis is characterized by pruritus or burning at the site of contact of an irritant or allergen. Lesions vary depending on the stage of response. In the acute stage erythema and oozing vesicles are common. Fungal infection typically affects scalp, trunk, limbs, face, groin or feet and is characterized by erythematous, scaling plaques. Cellulitis is characterized by diffuse, sharply defined, erythema. Red streaks run from the cellulitis toward regional lymph nodes. Scabies is characterized by minute vesicles and linear runs or burrows often found in digital webs, palms, wrists, gluteal folds, buttocks, and toes (Lommel & Jackson, pp. 236-237; Dains, et al., pp. 71-83).

26. **(d)** Topical corticosteroid agents are generally effective in the treatment of mild, uncomplicated contact dermatitis. Systemic corticosteroid therapy may be indicated for more severe episodes (Lommel & Jackson, p. 243).

27. **(b)** The characteristic lesion of Lyme disease (erythema migrans) is annular and erythematous with central pallor at the site of the tick bite. The lesion usually grows to 15 cm in diameter (range 3 to 68 cm). It typically appears from 3 to 32 days after the tick bite and is nonpruritic (Lommel & Jackson, p. 278).

28. **(d)** Characteristics of malignant melanoma include: A — asymmetry of borders, B — border irregularity or notching, C — color variation, and D — diameter greater than 6 mm. Malignant melanoma is seen in young, middle

age, and older adults. The most common form of skin cancer is basal cell carcinoma that often presents as a papule with rolled borders and a central umbilication or ulceration (Blackwell, pp. 493-494, 497).

29. **(c)** Risk factors for glaucoma include increasing age, family history of glaucoma, African-American race, diabetes mellitus, and myopia. The American Academy of Ophthalmology recommends glaucoma screening by an ophthalmologist for African-Americans who are age 20 to 39 every 3 to 5 years. Everyone age 40 to 64, regardless of race, should be screened every 2 to 4 years, and every 1 to 2 years beginning at age 65. Glaucoma screening with a Schiötz tonometer is relatively insensitive and nonspecific (DHHS, p. 321).

30. **(d)** Symptoms of viral conjunctivitis include gradual onset of unilateral (may become bilateral) scratchy sensation in the eye. There is no eye pain, vision changes, or photophobia. Examination of the eye reveals peripheral injection and a watery discharge. Allergic conjunctivitis is bilateral and the eyes are itchy. There is peripheral injection and a mucoid discharge. There is typically pain and photophobia with corneal abrasion. Subconjunctival hemorrhage is painless and without discharge. There is a splash of blood in the conjunctiva and sclera (Dains, et al., pp. 60-61).

31. **(a)** When the woman in an abusive situation is ready to open up, encouragement to discuss the abuse in specific and concrete terms is useful in helping her to validate her experience and to evaluate her level of danger. Asking the woman what she has done differently during the period of time that he has not been abusive implies that she does something to precipitate the abuse. Leaving is often a difficult process for the woman and, until she is ready and has safe plans, may not be the best thing for her to do. Although couple counseling is an option, it is often more beneficial when the abuse has been long term for the woman to seek counseling on her own first (Lowdermilk, et al., pp. 1230-1231; Rosenfeld, pp. 248-250).

32. **(c)** The cycle of violence has three phases: Phase 1 is the tension building state, phase 2 is the acute battering incident, and phase 3 is the honeymoon phase. The honeymoon phase is characterized by the abusive partner acting apologetic and remorseful. He may promise her that the battering will never occur again. When stress or other factors cause conflict and tension, the cycle is repeated (Lowdermilk, et al., p. 1227).

33. **(d)** Substance (including alcohol) dependence is defined as a maladaptive pattern of substance use, in the presence of at least three of seven elements, occurring at any time in the same 12 month period. One of these elements of dependence is a persistent desire to use the substance and/or unsuccessful efforts to cut down use. The other answers are elements of substance abuse rather than substance dependence. The person with alcohol dependence may exhibit elements of alcohol abuse (Nelson, p. 24).

34. **(b)** A central or abdominal pattern of body fat distribution in women is associated with type 2 diabetes and coronary heart disease. No strong association has been made with peripheral (lower body) fat distribution and these two obesity related diseases. Women typically demonstrate a peripheral body fat distribution pattern. Waist to hip ratio can be used to assess risk related to obesity. A ratio of > 0.8 indicates an increased risk (divide waist circumference at umbilicus by hip circumference at widest point). According to the medical classification of obesity the woman who is 20% over desirable weight and/or who has a body mass index of 25 would meet the definition of being overweight but not obese. According to the National Institutes of Health, the risk to health begins when body mass index exceeds 27 (Carlson, et al., pp. 459-460; Carr, et al., pp. 690-691).

35. **(a)** Moderate exercise is an important component of weight loss for women as it helps to increase lean body mass which in turn increases the basal metabolic rate. Moderate aerobic exercise has not been shown to cause an increase in appetite. Neither the American Heart Association nor the American College of Cardiology recommends routine screening by exercise testing in asymptomatic persons. They indicate that screening by exercise testing may be reasonable for persons with two or more cardiac risk factors prior to starting a vigorous exercise program. While it is important for this woman to discontinue smoking, this is not a contraindication to starting an exercise routine (DHHS, p. 414; Carlson, et al., p. 462).

36. **(d)** Depression is seen in about 50% of anorexia nervosa cases and even more frequently with bulimia nervosa. Alcohol/drug abuse and a lack of control are characteristic of bulimia nervosa but not anorexia nervosa; fear of loss of control predominates in anorexia nervosa. Amenorrhea is one of the diagnostic criteria for anorexia nervosa. Bulimia nervosa may lead to menstrual irregularities but usually not amenorrhea (Star, et al., sect. 14, pp. 32-33).

37. **(c)** The DSM-IV diagnostic criteria for a Major Depressive Episode includes five or more of a group of particular symptoms that present for a two week period and represent a change from previous level of function. One of the five symptoms *must* be either depressed mood or loss of interest or pleasure in most activities. The symptoms the woman describes are included in the diagnostic symptoms group as are feelings of worthlessness, excessive guilt and thoughts about dying or committing suicide (Rosenfeld, pp. 185-186).

38. **(d)** Serotonin reuptake inhibitors such as paroxetine usually have an energizing effect and may lead to insomnia if taken at night. Even when they are taken during the day they can still cause insomnia. Trazodone is a heterocyclic antidepressant that has a sedative effect so it is most beneficial to take it at night. These two groups of antidepressants are frequently used in combination as first-line treatment for major depression (Carlson, et al., p. 435; Carr, et al., pp. 734-735).

39. **(a)** Accident related injuries kill more children and adolescents than all other causes combined. Almost half of these injury related deaths are due to motor vehicle accidents. Anticipatory guidance for all individuals in this age group should include advice to always wear seat belts in the car. In addition, adolescents should be counseled to avoid drinking and driving and to avoid riding in a car driven by a person who has been drinking. Of course, counseling in relation to the other answer choices is also important, but they are not related to the leading cause of death for this age group (DHHS, pp. 149-152).

40. **(d)** According to the food guide pyramid, the minimum recommended servings for each food group are: Milk—2, meat—2, vegetables—3, fruit—3, and breads—6. The diet described includes milk—4, meat—3, vegetables—3, fruit—2 and breads—3 (DHHS, p. 403).

41. **(c)** The leading causes of death for women 50 to 64 years of age are coronary artery disease, breast, lung, colorectal and ovarian cancer, cerebrovascular disease and obstructive lung disease. ACOG guidelines recommend cholesterol and HDL screening every five years, mammography annually, annual fecal occult blood testing, and sigmoidoscopy every 3 to 5 years (ACOG, p. 246).

42. **(c)** Hypertension is defined as blood pressure of 140/90 mm Hg or greater at least three times on two separate occasions. Lifestyle changes for hypertension control recommended by the Joint National Committee on Prevention, Detection, Evaluation, and Treatment of High Blood Pressure include: Lose weight if overweight, limit daily alcohol intake to no more than one drink, increase aerobic physical activity to 30 to 45 minutes most days of the week, reduce sodium intake to no more than 100 mmol/dL, maintain adequate intake of dietary potassium, calcium and magnesium, and stop smoking. Estrogen replacement therapy is not indicated for a premenopausal woman (DHHS, pp. 188-191).

43. **(a)** A total cholesterol of 240 mg/dL has been demonstrated to double the risk of death from CHD as compared to a normal value of 200 mg/dL (ACOG p. 232).

44. **(d)** Women who are more than 30% overweight are more likely to develop heart disease even if it is their only risk factor. The use of estrogen replacement therapy after menopause may reduce the risk of heart disease by as much as 50%. Smoking is, of course, also a risk factor for the development of heart disease (Youngkin & Davis, pp. 706-707).

45. **(c)** Sharp, nonexertional chest pain of short duration is a symptom of mitral valve prolapse. Palpitations and diaphoresis may accompany the pain. Other symptoms may include anxiety and/or panic attacks. The diagnostic hallmark of mitral valve prolapse is a middle to late systolic click, a late systolic murmur, and an abnormally thickened, redundant mitral valve seen on echocardiogram. Often mitral valve prolapse is asymptomatic. It rarely progresses to mitral insufficiency (Hill & Geraci, pp. 29-30; Dains, et al., p. 100).

46. **(c)** An elevated TSH and a suppressed FT_4 are indicative of primary hypothyroidism. Periorbital edema is the only physical examination finding included in the possible answers that is associated with hypothyroidism (Youngkin & Davis, p. 758).

47. **(b)** The beginning of accelerated growth is usually the first sign of female puberty, but breast budding is the first recognized pubertal change. It is followed by the appearance of pubic hair and axillary hair. Peak growth velocity occurs about one year before menarche (Berek, et al., p. 774).

48. **(b)** Mononucleosis is most often a disease of young adults. Presentation is commonly a mild sore throat, low grade fever, malaise, anorexia, and fatigue. Physical findings often include pharyngeal exudate, petechiae on the palate, and cervical lymphadenopathy. Splenomegaly may also be present. The heterophil antibody blood test or monospot test is a test for mononucleosis. Group A β-hemolytic streptococcal pharyngitis is most common in children 5 to 15 years of age. It presents with acute onset of fever, sore throat and malaise. Pharyngeal exudate and cervical lymphadenopathy are common physical findings. Gonococcal pharyngitis is often asymptomatic. Physical findings of pharyngeal exudate and cervical lymphadenopathy may be present. A Tzanck smear may be done if there are lesions suggestive of herpes simplex (Dains, et al., pp. 27-28; Lommel & Jackson, pp. 39-40, 43).

49. **(a)** Risk factors for diabetes include being of Native American, Hispanic or African-American ethnicity, obesity, hypertension or hyperlipidemia, history of glucose intolerance, family history of parent or sibling with diabetes, and history of gestational diabetes or macrosomia (ACOG, p. 84).

50. **(a)** The presenting signs and symptoms are indicative of hyperthyroidism. Graves' disease comprises 70% of hyperthyroid cases and is seen most commonly in women 20 to 40 years of age. Subacute thyroiditis may also cause hyperthyroidism, but the thyroid is usually tender and the overlying skin warm and erythematous (Youngkin & Davis, p. 759; Blackwell, pp. 254).

51. **(a)** Propranolol is a beta-adrenergic blocking agent that may decrease the effectiveness of beta-adrenergic bronchodilators such as albuterol. Also, propranolol may potentiate the action of theophylline and lead to toxicity (Deglin & Vallerand, pp. 170, 179).

52. **(c)** Presenting symptoms and vital signs are indicative of bacterial pneumonia. Findings of consolidation associated with pneumonia would include increased vocal fremitus, presence of bronchophony, and dullness to percussion over affected lung areas (Dains, et al., p. 143).

53. **(c)** Daily prednisone use may alter immune function. Individuals with altered immune function may get false negative results with PPD testing. Multiple puncture tests such as the Tine test have been demonstrated to have a high

false negative rate and are not recommended for TB screening. Asthma, in itself, will not affect PPD test results (DHHS, p. 309; Pagana & Pagana, p. 1024).

54. **(b)** The CDC criteria for determining need for preventive therapy of TB is as follows: Consider treating individuals *without* risk factors in low incidence groups if they have an induration of 15 mm and are under 35 years of age; treat individuals *without* risk factors but in a high incidence group if they have induration of > 10 mm and are under 35 years of age; treat individuals *with* risk factors at all ages if they have induration of > 10 mm (or > 5 mm and recent TB contact, HIV infected or if have radiographic evidence of old TB). High incidence groups include foreign born persons from high prevalence countries, medically underserved low income populations, and residents of long term care facilities. Risk factors include HIV infection, recent (within past three months) contact with an infectious person, radiograph other than entirely normal, injection drug abuse, certain medical risk factors, and recent skin test conversion. Individuals who have received the BCG vaccine in the past may have a false positive. False negatives can occur with inactive vaccine and improper placement (DHHS, pp. 310-311).

55. **(b)** Risk factors for a complicated course include age over 65, altered mental status, suspicion of aspiration (due to her history of stroke), respiratory rate of 30 bpm or more, and temperature of 101° F with mental status changes (Ling, p. 246).

56. **(a)** Live vaccines, such as MMR may interfere with the response to the Mantoux test. The TB test should be delayed for 4 to 6 weeks after the MMR is administered (DHHS, p. 310).

57. **(d)** Positive screening tests such as the ELISA must be confirmed with a more specific supplemental test such as the Western blot. If confirmed by the supplemental test, a positive test result indicates that the individual is infected with HIV and is capable of transmitting the virus to others (CDC, p. 12).

58. **(d)** A glycosylated hemoglobin level or Hemoglobin A_{1c} provides an accurate long term index of the diabetic's average blood glucose level. As RBCs circulate, they combine some of their hemoglobin with some of the glucose in the bloodstream to form glycohemoglobin. This process is irreversible.

The amount of glycohemoglobin depends on the amount of glucose available in the bloodstream over the RBC's 120 day life span. Therefore, the glycosylated hemoglobin level reflects the average blood glucose level for the 100 to 120 days prior to the test (Pagana & Pagana, pp. 238-239).

59. **(b)** The CDC case definition for chronic fatigue syndrome includes specific fatigue criteria and four or more symptoms from a set of symptom criteria present for six months or more. These symptoms are sore throat, short term memory or concentration impairment, tender cervical or axillary lymph nodes, headaches of a new type, pattern or severity, unrefreshing sleep, post exertional malaise lasting more than 24 hours, multi-joint pain without swelling or inflammation, and muscle pain. In addition, the case definition includes specific exclusion criteria. There is no evidence of a hormonal relation in chronic fatigue syndrome. The syndrome does occur more commonly in women but not necessarily in the perimenopause (Houde & Kampfe-Leacher, pp. 30, 35-36).

60. **(b)** Counseling for both the individual with chronic fatigue syndrome and for family members may be helpful in coping with symptoms, psychological issues, and necessary lifestyle adjustments. While multivitamins have not been proven to cause a decrease in symptoms, in appropriate doses they are not harmful. A moderate exercise routine may be suggested at a level that does not increase fatigue. Recent studies have shown no beneficial effect of fluoxetine on any symptoms of chronic fatigue syndrome including depression (Houde & Kampfe-Leacher, pp. 46-48).

Gynecology

Beth Kelsey
Ann Salomone

Select one best answer to the following questions.

Questions 1 and 2 refer to the following scenario.

A 22-year-old female presents with a complaint of increased vaginal discharge, no itching, and an unpleasant odor. On examination a grayish white discharge is noted at the introitus and adhering to the vaginal walls. There is no erythema.

1. The most likely finding on a wet mount examination will be:

   a. Clue cells
   b. Pseudohyphae
   c. Trichomonads
   d. White blood cells

2. What is the CDC recommended treatment for this client?

   a. Doxycycline
   b. Metronidazole
   c. Ofloxacin
   d. Terconazole

3. A 65-year-old female presents with a complaint of intense itching in her vulvar area for the past month. She has not noticed any abnormal vaginal discharge. On examination, thick white plaques are noted in the vulvar area. There is no discrete mass noted. Initial management for this client should include:

   a. Biopsies of the affected area
   b. Patch testing for allergies
   c. Topical hydrocortisone cream
   d. Vaginal antifungal medication

4. A 20-year-old female presents with a complaint of swelling on one side of her labia. On examination, a 3 cm nontender cystic mass is noted lateral to the posterior vestibule. This is most likely a:

    a. Bartholin's duct cyst
    b. Skene's duct cyst
    c. Hidradenitis suppurativa
    d. Molluscum contagiosum

5. During a routine pelvic examination of a 24-year-old female who is not sexually active, the nurse practitioner finds a 4 cm, mobile, cystic ovarian mass. The client's LMP was three weeks ago. Appropriate management would include:

    a. Immediate referral for laparoscopy
    b. Initiation of antibiotics for salpingitis
    c. Ordering a CA-125 and pelvic ultrasound
    d. Repeating the pelvic examination in two months

Questions 6 and 7 refer to the following scenario.

A 26-year-old woman and her husband present at the clinic stating that they are having sexual problems. They have been married for three months and have not had sexual intercourse. They were reading a book about sexual problems and think that the problem is vaginismus.

6. An examination finding that would confirm that she has vaginismus would include:

    a. Localized tenderness and erythema at the introitus
    b. Involuntary vaginal spasm when a finger is inserted
    c. Presence of a transverse septum in the vagina
    d. Atrophy and friability of the vaginal epithelium

7. Treatment for vaginismus most often includes:

    a. Surgical intervention
    b. Behavioral therapy
    c. Tricyclic antidepressants
    d. Psychotherapy

8. Characteristics of normal vaginal secretions in a reproductive age woman include:

   a. Adherence to vaginal walls
   b. pH between 5.0 and 6.0
   c. Positive amine whiff test
   d. Presence of lactobacilli

Questions 9 and 10 refer to the following scenario.

A 24-year-old female was seen in the office and treated for her first yeast infection. Symptom relief was achieved. She calls the office three months later stating that she thinks she has another yeast infection as her symptoms are exactly the same as before.

9. Appropriate advice for this woman would include:

   a. Treatment of her and her partner to prevent reinfection
   b. Starting her on a treatment regimen for recurrent yeast infections
   c. Suggesting she try one of the over-the-counter yeast medications
   d. Encouraging her to consider testing for both diabetes and HIV infection

10. Six months later the same woman is seen in the office. She has a positive pregnancy test and another yeast infection. Recommended treatment for a yeast infection during pregnancy is:

   a. Clindamycin vaginal cream one applicator at bedtime for five days
   b. Clotrimazole 500 mg vaginal tablet, one tablet in a single application
   c. Fluconazole 150 mg oral tablet, one tablet in a single dose
   d. Terconazole vaginal cream one applicator at bedtime for seven days

Questions 11 and 12 refer to the following scenario.

A 23-year-old overweight nulliparous female presents with a history of periods every two to three months for the past two years. She has facial acne and is mildly hirsute. Her LMP was two months ago and her last sexual intercourse was three months ago. A pregnancy test today is negative.

11. The correct term for her menstrual pattern is:

   a. Amenorrhea
   b. Hypomenorrhea
   c. Oligomenorrhea
   d. Metrorrhagia

12. The most likely diagnosis for this client is:

    a. Androgen insensitivity syndrome
    b. Polycystic ovarian syndrome
    c. Premature ovarian failure
    d. Turner's syndrome

13. In which of these conditions would you expect a positive progesterone challenge test?

    a. Androgen insensitivity syndrome
    b. Polycystic ovarian syndrome
    c. Premature ovarian failure
    d. Turner's syndrome

Questions 14 and 15 refer to the following scenario.

A 40-year-old female presents with a complaint of heavy but regular periods occurring at her usual 27 to 28 day intervals. She states that her last period was very heavy and lasted for eight days. She has had no problems with cramping, but does feel some pressure in the pelvic area.

14. Expected pelvic examination findings with this client would include:

    a. Diffusely enlarged uterus
    b. Irregularly enlarged uterus
    c. Fixed retroverted uterus
    d. Prolapsed uterus

15. The correct terminology to describe her menstrual pattern is:

    a. Dysfunctional bleeding
    b. Menorrhagia
    c. Metrorrhagia
    d. Polymenorrhea

Questions 16, 17, and 18 refer to the following scenario.

A 32-year-old female presents with a complaint of menstrual cramps that start one or two days before her period and have gotten worse over the past six months. She has had occasional spotting a week before her period and has had increasing pain with sexual intercourse.

16. What is the most likely diagnosis for this client?

    a. Acute salpingitis
    b. Corpus luteum cyst
    c. Endometriosis
    d. Uterine fibroids

17. Expected pelvic examination findings for this client would include:

    a. Cervical motion tenderness
    b. Diffusely enlarged uterus
    c. Stenotic cervical os
    d. Nodules in the posterior fornix

18. A definitive diagnostic procedure for the above condition is:

    a. Culdocentesis
    b. Endometrial biopsy
    c. Laparoscopy
    d. Pelvic ultrasound

19. A 10-year-old female has recently developed breast buds. Which of the following statements would be true concerning this young girl?

    a. She is exhibiting signs of precocious puberty
    b. She will most likely start her periods in the next year
    c. She has most likely started her growth spurt
    d. She has probably developed pubic hair

20. Which of the following females, who has never had a period, would be considered to have primary amenorrhea?

    a. A 13-year-old who has no secondary sexual characteristics development
    b. A 14-year-old who has development of breast buds but no pubic hair
    c. A 15-year-old who has beginning breast development and some pubic hair
    d. A 16-year-old who has fully developed breasts and pubic hair

Questions 21, 22, and 23 refer to the following scenario.

An 18-year-old female, who is not sexually active, has never had a period. She has normal breast development and both pubic and axillary hair.

21. Possible causes for her primary amenorrhea include:

    a. Androgen insensitivity syndrome
    b. Asherman's syndrome
    c. Uterine agenesis
    d. Turner's syndrome

22. The genotype for this condition is:

    a. 45 X
    b. 46 XX
    c. 46 XY
    d. 47 XXY

23. A person with this condition would have:

    a. Absent or short vagina
    b. Endometrial adhesions
    c. Absent or streak ovaries
    d. Male gonads in the abdomen

Questions 24 and 25 refer to the following scenario.

A 45-year-old female, who had tubal sterilization two years ago, presents with a six month history of heavy, irregular periods every 24 to 30 days and lasting 8 to 10 days. Her LMP was two weeks ago. Pelvic examination reveals a normal size, non-tender uterus and normal adnexa.

24. Which one of the following tests would not be appropriate in the initial evaluation of this problem?

    a. Complete blood count
    b. Prolactin level
    c. Thyroid function test
    d. Transvaginal ultrasound

25. After an appropriate diagnostic evaluation, this client is determined to have dysfunctional uterine bleeding. Appropriate treatment might include:

    a. Bromocriptine
    b. Conjugated estrogen
    c. Medroxyprogesterone
    d. Prostaglandins

26. A 38-year-old female presents with menorrhagia and dysmenorrhea for the past

two years. Physical examination reveals a smooth, diffusely enlarged uterus which is slightly tender. The most likely diagnosis is:

    a. Adenomyosis
    b. Chronic pelvic infection
    c. Endometriosis
    d. Submucosal fibroids

27. Which of the following statements is true concerning primary dysmenorrhea?

    a. Age of onset is usually five or more years after menarche
    b. It is often associated with increased prostaglandin activity
    c. It is most often associated with anovulatory cycles
    d. Pain often begins 2 to 3 days before the period starts

28. A woman who will be taking a prostaglandin synthetase inhibitor (PGSI) for primary dysmenorrhea should be told to:

    a. Start the medication several days before the expected onset of her period
    b. Continue to take the medication through the last day of bleeding
    c. Try nonpharmaceutical measures for pain relief before taking medication
    d. Try a different one if the first PGSI is not effective

29. A 30-year-old female presents with complaints of monthly premenstrual symptoms that include anxiety, difficulty concentrating, bloating, and breast tenderness. She states that she experiences the same symptoms every month starting about one week before her period and resolving soon after her period starts. The most important part of this information in making a diagnosis of premenstrual syndrome is:

    a. Consistency of symptoms
    b. Number of symptoms
    c. Timing of symptoms
    d. Type of symptoms

30. The only therapy listed below that has consistently been shown through controlled research studies to be effective in the treatment of premenstrual syndrome is:

    a. Fluoxetine
    b. Oral contraceptives
    c. Progesterone suppositories
    d. Vitamin B_6

31. A 52-year-old female with a large uterine fibroid has been placed on leuprolide acetate, a GnRH agonist, to decrease the size of the tumor prior to surgical removal. Which of the following is a common side effect of this medication?

    a. Breast tenderness
    b. Headaches
    c. Nausea
    d. Hot flashes

32. An 18-year-old female complains of sharp, one sided, lower abdominal pain that occurs each month and lasts one to two days. She states that the pain seems to occur about two weeks after her period begins each month. A likely cause for this cyclic pain is:

    a. Rupture of the ovarian follicle
    b. Abnormal prostaglandin release
    c. Formation of a corpus luteum cyst
    d. Pelvic congestion syndrome

Questions 33 and 34 refer to the following scenario.

A 35-year-old female presents with no menses for the past three months. She has no galactorrhea and no symptoms of thyroid dysfunction. After ruling out pregnancy, a progesterone challenge test is administered. She has no withdrawal bleeding with this test. She does have withdrawal bleeding when both estrogen and progesterone are administered.

33. Which of the following laboratory tests is most appropriate as the next step in this client's evaluation?

    a. Cranial imaging—MRI
    b. FSH and LH levels
    c. Hysterosalpingography
    d. Serum estradiol level

34. Potential causes for this client's amenorrhea include:

    a. Androgen insensitivity syndrome
    b. Asherman's syndrome
    c. Hypothalamic dysfunction
    d. Polycystic ovarian syndrome

Questions 35 and 36 refer to the following scenario.

A nonpregnant 27-year-old female presents in your office with complaints of burning with urination and mild suprapubic discomfort for the past two days.

35. Which of the following would help you to determine whether she has cystitis or pyelonephritis?

    a. History of recurrent urinary tract infections
    b. Positive nitrites on a urine dipstick
    c. Presence of costovertebral angle tenderness
    d. > 10 WBC seen on urine microscopy

36. Laboratory tests and physical examination indicate that she has cystitis. She informs you that this is the fourth episode she has had in the past year and that they always seem to start a day or two after she has sexual intercourse. Instructions for using postcoital antibiotic prophylaxis include telling the patient to:

    a. Take the medication for three days after she has intercourse
    b. Take a one time dose just prior to or after intercourse
    c. Take medication for three days at the onset of any symptoms
    d. Take one dose of medication regularly one time each week

Questions 37 and 38 refer to the following scenario.

A 52-year-old female presents with a complaint of leaking urine. During questioning she admits that she does notice that it occurs when she laughs or coughs. She has had to give up her aerobics classes because she frequently leaks urine during the exercises.

37. What she is describing best fits the definition for:

    a. Stress incontinence
    b. Overflow incontinence
    c. Urge incontinence
    d. Functional incontinence

38. Treatment options that would be appropriate for the type of incontinence that this client is experiencing include:

    a. Antispasmodic agents
    b. Bladder retraining
    c. Intermittent catheterization
    d. Pelvic floor muscle exercises

39. A 24-year-old, single, sexually active female has a Pap smear report that indicates squamous metaplasia. Appropriate follow-up would include scheduling her for:

   a. An appointment to evaluate for cervical infection
   b. A repeat Pap smear in three to six months
   c. A return in one year for her next Pap smear
   d. An appointment for colposcopic evaluation

40. Which of the following statements about Pap smear specimen collection is true?

   a. All other cervical specimens should be obtained prior to obtaining the Pap smear specimen
   b. Excess mucus should be gently removed from the cervix with an applicator before obtaining the Pap smear specimen
   c. The bimanual examination should be performed prior to obtaining the Pap smear specimen
   d. The specimen should be applied thickly to the slide and then sprayed with fixative immediately

41. A 17-year-old sexually active female, who uses condoms for contraception, was seen two weeks ago for her first pelvic examination. At that time she had no complaints and her pelvic examination was normal. Two weeks later her test results have returned. Both the chlamydia and gonorrhea tests are negative. The Pap smear results are ASCUS favoring a reparative process. Appropriate management for a client with this Pap smear result would include:

   a. Repeating the Pap smear one week after her next period
   b. Repeating the Pap smear in four to six months
   c. Scheduling for colposcopic examination and biopsy
   d. Re-evaluating the client and treating any infection

42. Which of the following is a major advantage of loop electrosurgical excision procedure (LEEP) over either cryosurgery or laser vaporization for the treatment of preinvasive cervical lesions?

   a. Local anesthesia is rarely needed for the procedure
   b. There is less risk for postoperative hemorrhage
   c. Excised tissue provides a specimen for further evaluation
   d. There is less risk for postprocedure cervical stenosis

43. Which of the following is considered a risk factor for cervical cancer?

a. Smoking one pack of cigarettes per day
b. Uncircumcised sexual partner
c. Sexual partner with herpes infection
d. Use of talcum powder in the genital area

Questions 44 and 45 refer to the following scenario.

A 55-year-old female who currently is taking hormone replacement therapy says she has been reading about osteoporosis. She is concerned because she is fairly sedentary and she thinks she probably does not get enough calcium in her diet. A nutritional assessment shows that she gets about 500 mg of calcium through her diet on a daily basis.

44. Considering her current dietary calcium intake, the recommended calcium supplement for this client should be at least:

    a. 300 mg
    b. 500 mg
    c. 700 mg
    d. 1000 mg

45. This client states that she would like to increase her dietary intake of calcium but she doesn't use dairy products because she is lactose intolerant. Other good sources of calcium include:

    a. Chicken
    b. Citrus fruits
    c. Sardines
    d. Yellow vegetables

46. According to the current recommendations of several major medical authorities, bone density testing would be most appropriate:

    a. As a routine screening for a 35-year-old female with a family history of osteoporosis
    b. Prior to initiation of hormone replacement therapy for a 52-year-old obese, sedentary white female
    c. After a 52-year-old physically active African-American female makes the decision not to take hormone replacement therapy
    d. To assist a 50-year-old female smoker who is trying to decide if she wants to start hormone replacement therapy

47. For the menopausal woman who has a contraindication to estrogen use, a potential alternative treatment for hot flashes that is considered to be safe and effective is:

    a. Bellergal
    b. Clonidine
    c. Herbal ginseng
    d. Raloxifene

48. A 48-year-old client, currently taking low dose oral contraceptives, asks the nurse practitioner how she will know when it is time to switch to estrogen replacement therapy. An appropriate response would be to say that:

    a. She should discontinue oral contraceptives for three months so her FSH level can be measured
    b. She can discontinue oral contraceptives now and make the switch to estrogen replacement therapy
    c. She should have annual FSH levels drawn starting at age 50 on the last pill free day of her cycle
    d. She can stay on low dose oral contraceptives indefinitely as they will provide adequate estrogen

49. It would be appropriate to schedule an endometrial biopsy for a menopausal woman with an intact uterus:

    a. Annually if she is taking raloxifene as an alternative to estrogen replacement
    b. Annually if she is taking unopposed estrogen because she cannot tolerate progestins
    c. Three months after initiation of a continuous HRT regimen if she has any irregular bleeding
    d. One year after starting HRT if she continues to have bleeding during the hormone free days

50. When discussing the use of estrogen replacement for osteoporosis prevention with a client, the clinician should consider that:

    a. Estrogen replacement dosage should be the equivalent of at least 0.325 mg of conjugated estrogen
    b. There is no significant protection from bone loss if estrogen is started more than five years after menopause
    c. Transdermal administration of estrogen is less beneficial than oral administration in preventing bone loss

    d. Estrogen replacement should be continued for several years to reduce the risk of fractures

51. A 65-year-old woman currently on cyclic hormone replacement therapy is at your office for a routine annual examination. She states she has been healthy in the last year and she is having no problems with her HRT. On bimanual examination, a 4 cm nontender ovary is palpated. Appropriate management for this woman would include:

    a. Referring her to the gynecologist for further evaluation
    b. Discontinuing HRT and repeating the bimanual examination in two months
    c. Changing to a continuous HRT regimen and rechecking in two months
    d. Having her return in one year as this is a normal finding for a 65-year-old

Questions 52, 53, and 54 refer to the following scenario.

A 42-year-old female is at the clinic for a routine physical examination. She states that she has never had a mammogram because there is no breast cancer in her family. She also states that she does not know how to do a breast self-examination.

52. Which of the following information would be appropriate to share with this woman concerning risk factors for breast cancer?

    a. Over 50% of women who get breast cancer have a first degree relative who has had breast cancer
    b. The majority of women who get breast cancer do not have apparent risk factors
    c. One out of every 12 women in the United States will get breast cancer in her lifetime regardless of family history
    d. Other risk factors such as early menarche and late menopause are just as important as family history

53. As part of instructions on doing breast examination, the nurse practitioner advises the client to inspect her breasts with her arms raised above her head. This step is done to:

    a. Check for spontaneous nipple discharge
    b. More easily palpate axillary nodes
    c. Note any muscle weakness in the chest area
    d. Reveal changes in breast contour or symmetry

54. According to the latest American Cancer Society (ACS) recommendations, this 42-year-old client should:

    a. Have a baseline mammogram between age 40 and 45
    b. Start having annual mammograms now
    c. Start having annual mammograms when she is 50
    d. Have a mammogram every two years starting at age 50

55. For which of the following women would a breast ultrasound be most appropriate?

    a. A 25-year-old with a nontender, palpable mass
    b. A 30-year-old with nipple discharge from one breast
    c. A 40-year-old with breast pain and no palpable mass
    d. A 55-year-old with mammogram showing microcalcifications

Questions 56 and 57 refer to the following scenario.

A 30-year-old female presents with a complaint of a nipple discharge. Her LMP was two months ago, and she says it has not been unusual for her to skip periods for 2 to 3 months in the past year. She had a tubal sterilization two years ago after delivering her second child. Her pregnancy test today is negative.

56. If this client's nipple discharge is related to hyperprolactinemia, expected characteristics of the discharge would include its:

    a. Occurring in only one breast
    b. Occurring only with nipple stimulation
    c. Involving multiple ducts
    d. Having a yellow, sticky consistency

57. Additional history that would be pertinent in determining the potential cause for her hyperprolactinemia would include asking about:

    a. Symptoms of hyperthyroidism
    b. Use of tricyclic antidepressants
    c. Symptoms of premature ovarian failure
    d. Family history for diabetes mellitus

58. A 45-year-old female presents with spontaneous bloody nipple discharge from her left breast. On examination, no mass is noted and a bloody discharge is expressed from a single duct. The most likely diagnosis is:

    a. Breast carcinoma

   b. Duct ectasia
   c. Fat necrosis
   d. Intraductal papilloma

59. A 23-year-old female presents with a lump in her breast. On examination, a single, firm, nontender, mobile mass is palpated. The most likely diagnosis is:
   a. Breast carcinoma
   b. Fibroadenoma
   c. Fibrocystic change
   d. Galactocele

Questions 60 and 61 refer to the following scenario.

A 54-year-old woman has been scheduled for a modified radical mastectomy for breast cancer, and has been advised that she will probably be started on tamoxifen after the surgery.

60. In a modified radical mastectomy the:
   a. Breast, axillary nodes, and pectoralis major are removed
   b. Breast and a sampling of lymph nodes are removed
   c. Segment of breast and a sampling of lymph nodes are removed
   d. The tumor and a small amount of surrounding tissue are removed

61. When educating this client concerning the use of tamoxifen, it is important to tell her that:
   a. It should be taken for no more than six months after surgery
   b. Side effects of this medication include acne and hirsutism
   c. Use of this medication increases the risk for endometrial cancer
   d. It cannot be used if cancer cells are estrogen receptor positive

62. Which of the following is accurate regarding the use of mifepristone (RU486) for abortion?
   a. Misoprostol, a prostaglandin, is used with mifepristone to prevent heavy bleeding
   b. Mifepristone (RU486) works primarily as an antiprogesterone agent
   c. Mifepristone (RU486) has been shown to be effective for 2nd trimester termination
   d. Serious adverse reactions to mifepristone (RU486) have recently been reported

63. A 21-year-old female has a suction curettage abortion nine weeks after her LMP. She presents six days after the procedure with a complaint of heavy vaginal bleeding and moderate abdominal cramping for the past 48 hours. On examination her temperature is 99.6° F, blood is present in the vagina, and the cervical os is closed. The uterus is tender but firm. These findings are indicative of:

    a. Continuing intrauterine pregnancy
    b. Retained products of conception
    c. Postabortion syndrome
    d. Postabortal endometritis

64. Which of the following aspects of sexual functioning is least likely to be affected by the normal changes in a woman's body as she gets older?

    a. Amount of lubrication
    b. Duration of orgasms
    c. Intensity of orgasms
    d. Sexual desire or libido

Questions 65 and 66 refer to the following scenario.

A 30-year-old female presents at the emergency room stating that she was raped earlier that same evening. She appears anxious and smiles nervously while answering questions about the incident. Her breath smells of alcohol and her speech is slightly slurred. She states that her last consensual intercourse was about one week ago. She has not used birth control for the past year as she would like to get pregnant.

65. Appropriate documentation by the clinician who performs the sexual assault evaluation would include:

    a. The total number of sexual partners the victim has had
    b. Whether victim's emotional status seems appropriate
    c. The clinician's judgment of whether a rape occurred
    d. Activities of the victim after the rape occurred

66. Which of the following tests would not be routinely ordered as part of assessment of this sexual assault victim?

    a. Serologic test for HIV
    b. Urine pregnancy test
    c. Urine toxicology screen
    d. Pubic hair sampling

67. A 28-year-old woman presents for a routine checkup. She tells the clinician that her mother took DES when she was pregnant with her. She does not think she ever had any special tests because of the exposure to DES. Special tests to consider because of this client's DES exposure history include:

    a. Colposcopic examination
    b. Endometrial biopsy
    c. Mammogram
    d. Pelvic ultrasound

68. A 24-year-old female presents in the emergency room with temperature 102° F, blood pressure 80/40 mm Hg, diffuse macular erythema, and desquamation involving her fingers and toes. She has also had vomiting and diarrhea for the past 48 hours. The most likely diagnosis is:

    a. Acute allergic reaction
    b. Acute salpingitis
    c. Toxic shock syndrome
    d. Secondary syphilis

69. Which of the following is not an indication for colposcopic examination?

    a. Cellular changes associated with herpes
    b. Cervical leukoplakia
    c. Persistent cervical bleeding
    d. Baseline examination for women with HIV

70. Which of the following statements concerning endocervical polyps is true?

    a. The incidence is highest in women over 60-years-old
    b. Intermenstrual bleeding is a common symptom
    c. Polyps often represent a precancerous condition
    d. Dyspareunia is a frequent complaint with polyps

71. Which of the following occurs first in a normal menstrual cycle?

    a. Corpus luteum formation
    b. LH surge
    c. Ovulation
    d. Peak in progesterone level

72. The endometrial phase that corresponds with the luteal ovarian phase is the:

    a. Follicular phase

    b. Menstrual phase
    c. Proliferative phase
    d. Secretory phase

Questions 73 and 74 refer to the following scenario.

A couple has decided to use the fertility awareness method for contraception. They will be combining the use of basal body temperature (BBT), cervical changes, and the calendar method and plan to use abstinence during the woman's fertile days. She has regular periods that occur every 26 to 28 days.

73. This couple should be instructed to avoid sexual intercourse:

    a. For 48 hours after a rise of 0.4 degrees in her BBT
    b. From day 10 through day 20 of each menstrual cycle
    c. When the woman's cervix feels high in the vagina and soft
    d. From the end of her period until she has sticky cervical mucus

74. Other important information for this couple will include that the woman's ovum maintains the potential for fertilization for up to ____ hours, and once sperm is ejaculated into the vagina it can survive for up to ____ hours.

    a. 12 ; 24
    b. 24 ; 12
    c. 24 ; 72
    d. 48 ; 96

75. When fitting a woman for a diaphragm, it is important to remember that when correctly fitted it should:

    a. Allow a finger tip between it and the pubic arch
    b. Be small enough to allow for vaginal expansion
    c. Lie snugly over the pubic arch and under the cervix
    d. Provide firm tension against the vaginal walls

76. In making the choice of diaphragm type, the clinician might choose a flat spring diaphragm if the woman has:

    a. A large pubic arch notch
    b. Firm vaginal muscle tone
    c. A retroverted uterus
    d. A cystocele or rectocele

77. A woman using a diaphragm for birth control has sexual intercourse at 8:00 p.m. on Friday, 2:00 a.m. on Saturday, and 8:00 a.m. on Saturday. When can she safely remove her diaphragm for effective contraception, while minimizing problems related to leaving the diaphragm in for extended periods of time?

    a. 10 a.m. on Saturday
    b. 2 p.m. on Saturday
    c. 10 p.m. on Saturday
    d. 8 a.m. on Sunday

Questions 78 and 79 refer to the following scenario.

A 28-year-old female calls your office on Monday morning stating that the condom broke when she and her partner had sexual intercourse early Saturday afternoon. She is interested in postcoital contraception.

78. In discussing options with this client, it is important to explain that the latest she should wait before initiating hormonal postcoital contraception would be:

    a. Monday afternoon
    b. Monday evening
    c. Tuesday afternoon
    d. Wednesday morning

79. If she decides to take hormonal postcoital contraception and takes the initial dose at 10:00 a.m. on Monday, she will need to take her second dose at:

    a. 2:00 p.m. on Monday
    b. 6:00 p.m. on Monday
    c. 10:00 p.m. on Monday
    d. 10:00 a.m. on Tuesday

Questions 80 and 81 refer to the following scenario.

A three-week-postpartum woman who is breast feeding presents in your office to discuss her contraceptive options. Currently she is breast feeding on demand and is not providing any supplements. She plans to continue breast feeding for at least six months. She wants to know if she should restart her birth control pills or if she is protected from getting pregnant as long as she is breast feeding.

80. When counseling this woman concerning the lactational amenorrhea method of contraception, the nurse practitioner should tell her that:

a. The expected failure rate for this method of contraception is about 20%
b. This method is considered effective for only three months postpartum
c. The woman can rely on this method as long as she is amenorrheic
d. Another method should be used if the infant is sleeping through the night

81. She then asks you if she can restart birth control pills now as she wants to be sure that she does not get pregnant. The best response would be to tell her that:

a. Combination birth control pills are contraindicated while breast feeding
b. She can start her pills now and use a back up method for one month
c. She should wait until she has regular periods before restarting her pills
d. Progestin only pills would be a better option than combination pills

Questions 82 and 83 refer to the following scenario.

An 18-year-old female who has been on oral contraceptives for the past two years tells you that her dermatologist has given her oral tetracycline 500 mg b.i.d. for treatment of moderate inflammatory acne.

82. She should be advised that:

a. She should switch to a 50 mcg estrogen pill while on tetracycline
b. She should use a backup method for the first three weeks on tetracycline
c. Oral contraceptives may decrease the effectiveness of antibiotics
d. She should switch to a pill with a higher androgenic activity

83. The same client returns in six months and tells you that the dermatologist has recently started her on isotretinoin as her acne was not improving. She is thinking about quitting her pills in case they are causing her acne. She should be advised that:

a. She should use a barrier method of birth control while on isotretinoin
b. Discontinuing pills may cause her to have an exacerbation of acne
c. It is unlikely that birth control pills are causing her problem with acne
d. The effectiveness of her pills may be decreased by the use of isotretinoin

Questions 84 and 85 refer to the following scenario.

A 22-year-old female has one child and wants to wait about five years before having another child. She has been on oral contraceptives for the past three years without problems except that she frequently misses pills. She discontinued her pills about two months ago and is currently in the third day of her period. She is in the office today for a levonorgestrel insertion.

84. How soon after the levonorgestrel is inserted will she be able to safely rely on it for contraception?

   a. Within 24 hours
   b. After 48 hours
   c. In one week
   d. In one month

85. The next day she calls the clinic to say that she has a large bruise over her insertion site. You would advise her that:

   a. This is an expected occurrence after levonorgestrel insertion
   b. This may mean that one of the implants has broken
   c. This may be an indication of a reaction to the silicone
   d. This may be due to implants being inserted too superficially

Questions 86, 87, and 88 refer to the following scenario.

A 30-year-old woman is at the clinic for insertion of an IUD. She is currently having her period and has been using condoms consistently for contraception.

86. Which of the following should be performed first when preparing to insert her IUD?

   a. Application of a tenaculum to the cervix
   b. Cleansing of the cervix with antiseptic
   c. A bimanual examination
   d. Sounding of the uterus to determine size

87. Regarding the risk for infection with the insertion of an IUD, the clinician would want to keep in mind that:

   a. Inserting the IUD during menses has been shown to decrease the incidence of infection
   b. Prophylactic antibiotics have been shown to significantly decrease the incidence of infection
   c. The uterine cavity may remain unsterile for several months after IUD insertion
   d. The greatest risk for pelvic infection associated with use of the IUD is within one month following insertion

88. An IUD is inserted without problems. One year later the woman returns to the clinic and is found to be six weeks pregnant with the IUD still in place and the string visible. Counseling would include informing her that:

    a. There is a risk the baby will need to be delivered by C-section if the IUD is left in place
    b. There is an increased risk for preterm labor to occur if the IUD is left in place
    c. There is an increased risk of congenital anomalies due to the copper in the IUD
    d. There will be less risk of spontaneous abortion if the IUD is left in place than if removed

89. A 20-year-old female has been on phenytoin for several years to control her seizure disorder. She has no other problems and needs contraception. Of the following contraceptive methods, the best choice would be:

    a. Combination oral contraceptives
    b. Medroxyprogesterone acetate injections
    c. Levonorgestrel implants
    d. Progestin-only pills

90. The characteristic most often associated with a woman who regrets having had a tubal sterilization is:

    a. Having a change in marital status
    b. Total number of children
    c. Procedure immediately postpartum
    d. Younger age at time of procedure

91. A couple who is considering a vasectomy asks you how soon after the procedure they can discontinue using another form of contraception. The appropriate response would be to say that:

    a. Another method of contraception should be continued for three months
    b. The procedure is effective immediately so other contraception is not needed
    c. He should have three negative sperm counts before he is considered sterile
    d. Viable sperm may remain in the vas deferens until about 20 ejaculations

92. A woman has missed two pills in the third week of her pill package. Today is

Thursday and she normally starts her next pack on a Tuesday. In addition to advising this woman to use a backup method for seven days, she should be instructed to:

    a. Finish the current pack and start her new pack as usual
    b. Take two pills each day for the next two days, then continue pills as usual
    c. Continue the current pack until Sunday, then start a new pack
    d. Finish the third week of her pack, then start a new pack immediately

93. A 17-year-old female has been on oral contraceptives for one year without problems. In the last two months she has had some spotting. She has missed no pills and is on no other medications. Initial management should include:

    a. Advising her to return if spotting continues in the next cycle
    b. Changing her pills to a type with a better endometrial activity
    c. Performing a pelvic examination and tests for cervical infections
    d. Encouraging her to consider a different method of birth control

94. An advantage of the female condom is:

    a. It can be used with a male condom for added protection
    b. It can be used for repeated acts of intercourse
    c. It is made of polyurethane which is stronger than latex
    d. It is less expensive than most male condoms

95. A 20-year-old female who is 30% overweight is at the clinic to receive her first medroxyprogesterone acetate (DMPA) injection. Which of the following is true with regard to administering DMPA to this woman?

    a. She may need a larger dose than the usual 150 mg
    b. She should return for repeat injections every two months
    c. You should massage the injection site well to assure absorption
    d. You should choose a site that assures a deep IM injection

96. Progestin-only pill users should be instructed:

    a. To use a backup method for 48 hours if they are more than three hours late taking a pill
    b. To throw away the pack and start a new one if two pills are missed in the third week of a pack
    c. That ovulation is unlikely to occur with this method if pills are taken at the same time each day

d. That if a period is missed when using progestin-only pills, a pregnancy test should be done

97. A woman who has been managed with medroxyprogesterone acetate injections for nine months is one week late for her fourth injection. She states that the last time she had sexual intercourse was one week ago. Appropriate management would be:

a. Advising her to use condoms and return at her next menses for an injection
b. Giving the injection and advising her to return if she has no menses in the next month
c. Performing a sensitive pregnancy test and giving the injection if the test is negative
d. Starting her on oral contraceptives and giving the injection when she has her period

98. Which of the following is appropriate instruction when teaching use of the male condom?

a. Unroll the condom to check for holes before placing it on the penis
b. Be sure the rolled rim is on the outside when putting the condom on
c. Do not remove the condom until after the penis loses its erection
d. Do not use a condom that is more than one year past manufacture date

99. When comparing perfect use failure rates and typical use failure rates, the greatest difference between the two would be seen with which of the following methods?

a. Diaphragm
b. IUD
c. Levonorgestrel
d. Tubal sterilization

100. Noncontraceptive benefits of oral contraceptives include a decrease in the risk of:

a. Breast cancer
b. Cervical cancer
c. Colon cancer
d. Ovarian cancer

101. A normal semen analysis would show:

a. Sperm count 5 million/mL, motility of 60%, and morphology of 40% normal
b. Sperm count 15 million/mL, motility of 60%, and morphology of 30% normal
c. Sperm count 25 million/mL, motility of 50%, and morphology of 60% normal
d. Sperm count 50 million/mL, motility of 40%, and morphology of 40% normal

102. Which of the following statements concerning hysterosalpingography is correct?

a. It is usually performed 1 to 2 days after ovulation
b. It may be therapeutic as well as diagnostic
c. It involves transabdominal injection of dye into the uterus
d. It provides for direct visualization of the fallopian tubes

103. Varicoceles may cause infertility by:

a. Decreasing the sperm count
b. Causing retrograde ejaculation
c. Causing antibody formation
d. Causing erectile dysfunction

104. A 29-year-old female presents for her annual examination. She relates that she and her partner stopped using contraception the previous month and desire to start a family. She has several questions related to fertility awareness and the most optimum time to achieve pregnancy. You advise her that she is most fertile when her cervical mucus is:

a. Clear, watery, and stretchy, at the time it is primarily under the effect of estrogen
b. Clear, watery, and stretchy, at the time it is primarily under the influence of progesterone
c. Opaque, thick, and sticky, at the time it is primarily under the influence of estrogen
d. Opaque, thick and sticky, at the time it is primarily under the influence of progesterone

105. Instructions for the woman who is going to have a postcoital test include:

a. Abstaining from intercourse for 48 hours before the test
b. Coming to the office within 48 hours after intercourse

    c. Coming to the office within 48 hours after a positive LH test

    d. Having intercourse within 48 hours after a rise in BBT

106. Clomiphene citrate works as a/an:

    a. Dopamine receptor agonist that decreases prolactin levels

    b. Estrogen receptor agonist that enhances gonadotropin secretion

    c. Gonadotropin that stimulates ovarian follicular development

    d. Gonadotropin releasing hormone that stimulates estradiol secretion

107. A couple presents to you shortly after their marriage. The husband had a vasectomy three years ago after the birth of his last child. They are seeking information on the success rate of vasectomy reversals as they would like to have a child together. Which of the following reflects correct information?

    a. The success rate for a reversal is directly dependent on the man's current age

    b. Pregnancy rates following vasectomy reversal are generally 50% or greater

    c. He has probably developed significant antisperm antibodies since his vasectomy

    d. There is an increased risk of birth defects in pregnancies occurring after a reversal

108. Which of the following couples would be considered to have secondary infertility?

    a. The husband has fathered a child in a previous marriage but the current couple has been unable to conceive after trying for 12 months

    b. The couple has been able to conceive, but the woman has been unable to produce a live birth

    c. The couple has previously conceived but is now unable to achieve a pregnancy after trying for 12 months

    d. One member of the couple has been shown through testing to be fertile and the other has been shown to be infertile

Questions 109 and 110 refer to the following scenario.

109. A client presents with a history of vaginal discharge, dysuria, and postcoital bleeding. Physical examination reveals an erythematous, friable cervix. Urinalysis is within normal limits. Wet mount examination reveals many WBCs. Gram stain reveals gram negative diplococcus. Your presumptive diagnosis is:

    a. Gonorrhea

    b. Trichomoniasis

    c. Herpes cervicitis

    d. Chlamydia

110. Based on your diagnosis, the CDC recommended treatment for this infection would be:

    a. Ceftriaxone 125 mg IM plus doxycycline 100 mg p.o. b.i.d. for seven days

    b. Metronidazole 2 grams p.o. once

    c. Acyclovir 200 mg p.o. five times a day for seven days

    d. Azithromycin 1 gram p.o. once

Questions 111 and 112 refer to the following scenario.

111. A client presents with several small (1 to 5 mm in size) dome-shaped, waxy papules with umbilicated centers. They are located on her thighs and lower abdomen and do not itch. A likely diagnosis is:

    a. Acne vulgaris

    b. Erythema nodosum

    c. Folliculitis

    d. Molluscum contagiosum

112. Based on the above diagnosis, treatment recommendations include:

    a. Advising the client that the lesions are self-limiting and resolve spontaneously

    b. Applying tretinoin cream to the affected area twice a day for 7 to 14 days

    c. Instructing the client to apply hot soaks and then express the core material

    d. Excision and drainage of the lesions followed by erythromycin for 7 to 14 days

113. Which of the following statements concerning recurrent herpes is true?

    a. Recurrences during pregnancy should be treated with valacyclovir

    b. Systemic symptoms are uncommon during recurrent episodes

    c. Topical acyclovir is as effective as oral acyclovir for recurrent episodes

    d. Transmission of the virus is unlikely to occur during the prodromal phase

114. A Tzanck preparation may be used in the diagnosis of:

a. Antisperm antibodies
b. Herpes simplex
c. Syphilis
d. Tubal occlusion

115. A client who was treated the previous day with benzathine penicillin G for early syphilis calls to report that her muscles ache and she has a fever. Appropriate actions would include:

    a. Advising her to tell all future health care providers about this reaction
    b. Consulting a physician about additional tests for possible neurosyphilis
    c. Instructing her to go to the hospital as this may be an allergic reaction
    d. Recommending that she take acetaminophen for relief of her symptoms

116. A 26-year-old client was successfully treated for syphilis one year ago. She has remained abstinent since that time and you can be fairly certain that she has not become reinfected. Which of the following serologic test results would you expect at this time?

    a. RPR reactive, FTA-ABs negative
    b. RPR non-reactive, FTA-ABs negative
    c. RPR non-reactive, FTA-ABs positive
    d. RPR reactive, FTA-ABs positive

117. A 22-year-old female presents with complaint of lower abdominal pain since her period ended two days ago. She has had a new sexual partner in the past two months and does not use condoms. On examination you find that she has cervical motion tenderness. You are concerned that she may have pelvic inflammatory disease. To meet the CDC's minimum criteria for empiric treatment of pelvic inflammatory disease she must also have:

    a. An oral temperature of >101° F and mucopurulent cervicitis
    b. A positive test for cervical infection and an adnexal mass
    c. Lower abdominal tenderness and adnexal tenderness
    d. Mucopurulent cervicitis and an elevated WBC count

118. An 18-year-old female presents to your STD clinic with a white, crater appearing lesion on her labia minora. She states it began a week ago as a "pimple" and is not painful. Your Darkfield examination is positive. Treatment would include:

    a. Acyclovir 200 mg five times a day for 7 to 10 days
    b. Benzathine penicillin G 2.4 million units IM

   c. Cephalexin 250 mg three times a day for 7 to 14 days
   d. Triple antibiotic ointment applied three times a day

119. A client presents today for an examination with complaints of dysuria, vaginal discharge, and itching. She states that the symptoms were worse just before her period but she thinks they are coming back. Her partner has been away for two months so she has not been sexually active in a while. You obtain a wet mount which demonstrates a pH of 4.0, few WBCs, and pseudohyphae. You prescribe:

   a. Terconazole vaginal cream
   b. Metronidazole vaginal gel
   c. Clindamycin 2% vaginal cream
   d. Metronidazole 2 grams by mouth

120. A 22-year-old female comes to the office because she has noticed "bumps around her vagina." Your examination indicates that these are external genital warts. You would want to explain to her that:

   c. Her partner needs a test for subclinical infection
   b. She should have a Pap smear every six months
   c. There is no therapy that will eliminate the HPV virus
   d. You cannot start treatment until you have her Pap results

121. Common presenting symptoms and physical findings with infection caused by *Haemophilus ducreyi* include:

   a. A single, painful genital ulcer with inguinal lymphadenopathy
   b. Painless ulcerative lesions without regional lymphadenopathy
   c. Multiple, nonpruritic condyloma lata in the anogenital area
   d. Painful ulcers on mucous membranes and general lymphadenopathy

122. A 28-year-old female presents with the complaint of intense vaginal itching, especially at night and after intercourse. She complains of a "bad smell" especially after intercourse. Pelvic examination reveals erythema and frothy, yellow-green vaginal discharge. She relates that her partner has occasional symptoms of urethritis by history. You suspect:

   a. Bacterial vaginosis
   b. Chlamydia
   c. Gonorrhea
   d. Trichomoniasis

Answers and Rationales

1. **(a)** The most likely diagnosis for this client is bacterial vaginosis. Characteristics of this infection include an increased, malodorous vaginal discharge. There is usually no itching or erythema. The discharge is typically grayish white, is present at the introitus, and adheres to the vaginal walls. Clue cells are epithelial cells stippled with bacteria that obscure the cell border. This is a classic finding with bacterial vaginosis. Other findings include a vaginal discharge, pH > 4.5, and release of an amine (fishy) odor when KOH 10% is applied to the discharge (Youngkin & Davis, p. 268).

2. **(b)** The CDC recommended treatment for bacterial vaginosis in nonpregnant women is metronidazole 500 mg orally twice daily for seven days. The recommended regimen for pregnant women is metronidazole 250 mg orally three times a day for seven days (CDC, pp. 72-73).

3. **(a)** Several vulvar dystrophies occur more commonly in postmenopausal women. Biopsies are required to evaluate the presence of atypia or malignancy. Vulvar pruritus is one of the common presenting symptoms of vulvar cancer. A mass is common but not always present. Vulvar lesions with cancer may be fleshy, ulcerated, leukoplakic, or warty in appearance (Berek, et al., pp. 387, 1234).

4. **(a)** The Bartholin's gland ducts are located bilaterally at approximately 5 o'clock and 7 o'clock at the vaginal introitus. These ducts may become obstructed causing cyst formation. These cysts are usually not tender unless there is infection present (Havens, et al., p. 43).

5. **(d)** During the reproductive years most ovarian masses are benign. Follicular cysts, corpus luteum cysts, and theca lutein cysts are all benign, functional cysts which do not usually cause symptoms or require surgery. Follicular cysts are the most common and they are rarely greater than 8 cm in size. They are usually found incidental to pelvic examination and resolve on their own in 1 to 2 months. Pelvic ultrasound evaluation would not necessarily be inappropriate, but there is no indication for CA-125 with this client (Berek, et al., pp. 361-363).

6. **(b)** Vaginismus is a condition in which there is an involuntary spasm or contraction of the pubococcygeal muscle when a woman either anticipates or

experiences attempted entry of the vagina by a penis or other object such as a finger or speculum (Rosenfeld, p. 285).

7. **(b)** Psychotherapy and medications are usually not necessary for treatment of vaginismus. Surgical intervention is not indicated. Behavioral therapy is indicated to help the woman learn to voluntarily relax the involved muscles and progressively insert larger objects (1 finger, 2 fingers, etc.), and is usually successful (Rosenfeld, p. 286).

8. **(d)** Characteristics of normal vaginal secretions include a pH of 3.8 to 4.2, presence of epithelial cells, lactobacilli, and a variety of aerobic and anaerobic bacteria. Normal vaginal secretions pool in the posterior fornix and do not adhere to the vaginal walls (Mishell, et al., p. 625).

9. **(c)** Self medication with over-the-counter preparations is an acceptable option for women who have been diagnosed previously with a yeast infection and who have a recurrence of the same symptoms. If symptoms persist after using an over-the-counter preparation, or if symptoms recur within two months, clinical evaluation is indicated. Treatment of asymptomatic sex partners is not recommended. Because this is only the second yeast infection this woman has had, it would not meet the definition for recurrent yeast infection which is four or more episodes annually. There is no indication for HIV infection or diabetes testing in this situation (CDC, p. 77-78).

10. **(d)** Only the topical azoles should be used to treat pregnant women with yeast infections. Many experts recommend seven days of therapy during pregnancy rather than one of the shorter regimens (CDC, p. 78).

11. **(c)** Oligomenorrhea is infrequent, irregular episodes of bleeding usually occurring at intervals of more than 35 days (Berek, et al., p. 159).

12. **(b)** Polycystic ovarian syndrome is characterized by oligomenorrhea or amenorrhea, infertility, hirsutism, and obesity. Diagnostic criteria include hyperandrogenism and chronic anovulation. An elevated LH:FSH ratio is frequently, but not always, present. Cystic ovarian changes are usually present (Berek, et al., p. 837).

13. **(b)** A positive progesterone challenge test (withdrawal bleed) indicates the presence of endogenous estrogen and an intact endometrium in an individual with amenorrhea. Polycystic ovarian syndrome is the only answer choice in which both of these are present (Youngkin & Davis, p. 142).

14. **(b)** An enlarged, irregular uterus is an expected examination finding in the woman with uterine leiomyomas (fibroids). Leiomyomas may cause menorrhagia (heavy and/or prolonged periods occurring at regular intervals). Pelvic heaviness, discomfort, or pressure are often described (Youngkin & Davis, p. 337).

15. **(b)** As described in number 14, the definition of menorrhagia is regular episodes of bleeding that are excessive in amount and duration (Berek, et al., p. 159).

16. **(c)** Classic symptoms of endometriosis include secondary dysmenorrhea that is progressive, dyspareunia with deep penetration, and infertility. Premenstrual spotting is another common symptom (Youngkin & Davis, p. 315; Mishell, et al., p. 523).

17. **(d)** Signs of endometriosis on pelvic examination include nodularity in the cul-de-sac or along the uterosacral ligaments, which are located posterior to the uterus. The uterus may be fixed in a retroverted position (Mishell, et al., p. 524; Berek, et al., p. 891).

18. **(c)** Laparoscopy with biopsy of visible endometrial implants is currently the only definitive method of diagnosing endometriosis (Mishell, et al., pp. 524-525).

19. **(c)** Generally, accelerated growth is the first sign of puberty, followed by breast budding, then appearance of pubic hair, peak growth velocity, and menarche. This sequence of pubertal development generally takes 4.5 years (Berek, et al., p. 772; Youngkin & Davis, pp. 47-49).

20. **(d)** Primary amenorrhea is defined as the absence of menses by 16 years of age in the presence of normal secondary sexual characteristics or by age 14 when there is no visible secondary sexual characteristic development (Berek, et al., p. 809).

21. **(c)** Primary amenorrhea in association with normal breast development and normal pubic and axillary hair growth is often associated with uterine agenesis. This is the second most frequent cause of primary amenorrhea. The individual with androgen insensitivity syndrome will also have primary amenorrhea. Breast development occurs but there is little or no pubic or axillary hair. The female with Turner's syndrome has no secondary sexual characteristic development. Asherman's syndrome is characterized by scarring or adhesions in the intrauterine cavity. This is usually the result of uterine surgical procedures or pelvic infection. This would be an unlikely cause for an 18-year-old who has never had a period and is not sexually active (Mishell, et al., pp. 1049-1053).

22. **(b)** The individual with uterine agenesis has a normal female karyotype of 46XX. The individual with androgen insensitivity syndrome has a male karyotype of 46XY. 45X is seen with Turner's syndrome. 47XXY is seen with Klinefelter's syndrome in males (Mishell, et al., pp. 1049-1051).

23. **(a)** The individual with complete uterine agenesis will have a shortened or absent vagina. She will have normal ovaries. Endometrial adhesions are seen with Asherman's syndrome. The individual with Turner's syndrome will have absent or streak ovaries. The individual with Androgen insensitivity syndrome will have male gonads in the abdomen (Mishell, et al., pp. 1048-1053).

24. **(b)** Hyperprolactinemia is generally associated with amenorrhea or oligomenorrhea along with galactorrhea. The complete blood count with differential and platelet count can determine if anemia is present. Also, abnormalities may indicate the need for further evaluation for possible blood dyscrasias or thrombocytopenia. Thyroid function tests may reveal hypothyroidism, which is one of the more common systemic causes for abnormal uterine bleeding. Transvaginal ultrasound may be ordered to measure endometrial thickness and to look for endometrial polyps and submucous leiomyomas (Youngkin & Davis, pp. 145-146; Mishell, et al., pp. 1030-1031).

25. **(c)** Treatment options for chronic dysfunctional uterine bleeding include low dose oral contraceptives, medroxyprogesterone acetate, prostaglandin synthetase inhibitors, D&C, endometrial ablation, and hysterectomy. Conjugated estrogen may be administered intravenously or orally for treatment of acute dysfunctional bleeding (Youngkin & Davis, pp. 146-148).

26. **(a)** Adenomyosis is the growth of endometrial tissue in the myometrium. Dysmenorrhea may begin up to one week before menses and persist until after the period is over. Heavy bleeding is also associated with adenomyosis. Pelvic examination often reveals a diffusely enlarged, smooth uterus that is tender especially at the time of menses (Berek, et al., p. 412).

27. **(b)** Primary dysmenorrhea is menstrual pain without related pathology. The cause of primary dysmenorrhea is increased prostaglandin production in the endometrium. Onset is usually within one to two years of menarche when ovulatory cycles are established. Pain usually begins a few hours prior to or just after the onset of the period and may last as long as 48 to 72 hours (Berek, et al., p. 410).

28. **(a)** The client should try one PGSI for 2 to 4 cycles beginning several days before the expected start of her menses. If she does not get pain relief, it is reasonable to try another PGSI from a different pharmacological group (e.g. naproxen sodium versus ibuprofen). The newer prostaglandin synthetase inhibitors have a rapid onset of action so there is no need to start them several days prior to menses. Primary dysmenorrhea typically does not last throughout the entire period, and medication may be discontinued when no longer needed. While nonpharmaceutical measures such as heat application may be helpful, the prostaglandin synthetase inhibitors will be less effective if one waits very long after cramping starts to take the medication. Nonpharmaceutical measures may be helpful in combination with PGSI use (Youngkin & Davis, pp. 150-151).

29. **(c)** The main diagnostic criteria for PMS are that the symptoms begin in the luteal phase of the menstrual cycle and that there is a symptom free period starting within a few days of onset of menses (Blackwell, p. 503; Youngkin & Davis, p. 154).

30. **(a)** Fluoxetine has been shown in double-blind, placebo-controlled studies to be effective in treating the symptoms of PMS. Study results are conflicting for vitamin B_6, and women with PMS have not been shown to have a vitamin B_6 deficiency. Most studies using oral contraceptives have not shown a beneficial effect in relief of PMS symptoms. Double-blind, placebo-controlled studies with progesterone suppositories have not shown this therapy to be effective (Blackwell, pp. 506, 511-512; Youngkin & Davis, pp. 156-157).

31. **(d)** GnRH agonists such as leuprolide acetate act by causing a hypoestrogenic state in the woman. Side effects are similar to those experienced with menopause including hot flashes. Reversible bone loss may also occur with the use of this medication so it is only recommended for short term use (Berek, et al., p. 374).

32. **(a)** Midcycle pelvic pain is often associated with rupture of the ovarian follicle at the time of ovulation. This is called mittelschmerz (Berek, et al., p. 403).

33. **(b)** The absence of a withdrawal bleed after a progesterone challenge, but occurrence of bleeding after estrogen and progesterone are administered, suggests that the woman has inadequate endogenous estrogen production but an intact endometrium and outflow tract. Hypoestrogenism may result from problems anywhere in the hypothalamic-pituitary-ovarian axis. Elevated FSH and LH indicate that the problem is ovarian. Normal or low FSH and LH indicate that the problem is either in the hypothalamus or pituitary gland. A prolactin level may be indicated if not already obtained, and cranial imaging with CT or MRI may be considered if the FSH and LH are normal or low. An estradiol level is not necessary as hypoestrogenism has already been established, and a hysterosalpingography is not needed as an intact endometrium and outflow tract have been established (Berek, et al., pp. 826-827).

34. **(c)** Hypothalamic dysfunction results in differing levels of hypoestrogenism depending on the severity of the dysfunction. Hypothalamic dysfunction may be caused by chronic disease, anorexia nervosa, stress, excessive exercise, malnutrition, or rarely, an anatomic lesion. The individual with androgen insensitivity syndrome would have primary amenorrhea. Although she may have some withdrawal bleeding with Asherman's syndrome, the fact that she has had no menses, or even spotting for three months, makes this less likely. The individual with polycystic ovarian syndrome, will have a withdrawal bleed with a progesterone challenge (Berek, et al., p. 827).

35. **(c)** Costovertebral tenderness is usually present with pyelonephritis. It would not be present with cystitis (Dains, et al., pp. 234-235).

36. **(b)** Taking the antibiotic 30 minutes before or after intercourse is an option for women who have recurrent urinary tract infections directly related to sexual intercourse. Frequency of intercourse must be considered. Antibiotics

that can be considered include nitrofurantoin and trimethoprim/sulfamethoxazole (Youngkin & Davis, p. 854).

37. **(a)** Stress incontinence is the involuntary loss of urine during activities that increase intra-abdominal pressure such as laughing, coughing, and jumping. Urge incontinence is involuntary loss of urine associated with a sudden, strong urge to void. Overflow incontinence is a result of urinary retention with bladder distention and overflow of urine. Functional incontinence results from medically reversible causes such as delirium, infection, medications, and restricted mobility (Berek, et al., pp. 630, 639, 650, 654).

38. **(d)** Nonsurgical treatment for stress incontinence usually involves efforts to enhance the ability of the pelvic floor muscles to compensate for increased intra-abdominal pressure. These include muscle strengthening exercises, improving estrogen status, electrical stimulation of the muscles, and use of alpha-adrenergic stimulants. Bladder retraining and antispasmodics are used in treatment of urge incontinence. Intermittent catheterization may be used with bladder retention (Berek, et al., pp. 643-645, 652-653, 655).

39. **(c)** Squamous metaplasia is a normal process whereby cervical columnar epithelium is transformed into squamous epithelium. The area where this occurs is called the transformation zone (Mashburn & Scharbo-DeHaan, p. 115).

40. **(b)** If excess cervical mucus is present, it should be removed gently with a large cotton tipped applicator prior to obtaining the Pap smear specimen. To avoid contamination with blood, the Pap smear should be performed before other cervical sampling such as tests for chlamydia and gonorrhea. The Pap smear specimen should be applied to the glass slide in a thin layer and then sprayed immediately with fixative. The bimanual examination should be performed after the speculum examination to avoid contamination of the cervix with lubricant (DHHS, pp. 266-267).

41. **(b)** The recommended follow-up of a first time ASCUS Pap result favoring a reparative process is to repeat the Pap smear every 4 to 6 months for two years. If there is another abnormal Pap result during this follow-up period, colposcopic evaluation is indicated (Mashburn & Scharbo-DeHaan, pp. 127-128).

42. **(c)** A major advantage of LEEP is that it is not a destructive technique, so the excised tissue is suitable for further histologic examination. Both cryosurgery and laser vaporization destroy the transformation zone so a specimen is not available for further diagnostic evaluation (Youngkin & Davis, p. 356).

43. **(a)** Several studies have demonstrated an increased risk of cervical cancer among smokers. Potential mechanisms of connection between smoking and cervical cancer include nicotine and cotinine having a direct effect on cervical mucus, the oncogenicity of HPV being enhanced by tobacco smoke, and smoking causing local immunosuppression within the cervix. The other three choices have not been shown to increase the risk for cervical cancer (Brinton, pp. 9-10).

44. **(b)** The recommended daily calcium intake for the postmenopausal woman under 65-years-old, who is taking estrogen replacement, is 1000 mg. This woman would need a 500 mg supplement. Postmenopausal women not on estrogen replacement and all women 65 and older need 1500 mg of calcium daily (Millonig, p. 78; DHHS, p. 405).

45. **(c)** Good nondairy sources of calcium include sardines, salmon, broccoli, kale, collard greens, and tofu (Krummel & Kris-Etherton, p. 188).

46. **(d)** Bone density testing may be useful when the results will help a menopausal woman, with osteoporosis risk factors, who is trying to make a decision about whether or not she will use hormone replacement therapy. The information might also help the clinician in deciding on recommendations when weighing any risks versus benefits for an individual woman. Bone density testing is not currently recommended for routine screening in premenopausal women. Bone density testing would not be indicated for the woman who has made the decision to start HRT or for the low risk woman (African-American, physically active) who has made her decision not to take HRT (DHHS, pp. 456-457; Berek, et al., pp. 994-995).

47. **(b)** Clonidine, an antihypertensive drug used in low dosages, has been shown to be effective in relieving hot flashes. Bellergal may relieve hot flashes, but has sedative effects and is habit forming. Herbal ginseng is a potent

source of plant estrogen and should be not be used if the woman has contraindications to the use of estrogen. Hot flashes are a common side effect of raloxifene (Millonig, pp. 35-36; Murphy, p. 186).

48. **(c)** Women taking oral contraceptives may not experience the symptoms that indicate menopause is occurring. It is recommended that women taking oral contraceptives should start having annual FSH levels at age 50. To prevent an inaccurate result, the specimen should be drawn on day 6 or 7 of the pill free week (Speroff & Darney, p. 313; Hatcher, et al., p. 79).

49. **(b)** Women who still have a uterus and are taking unopposed estrogen should have annual endometrial evaluation because of the increased risk for endometrial hyperplasia or cancer. Raloxifene does not have an estrogen like effect on the endometrium, so there is no increased risk for endometrial hyperplasia or cancer and no need for annual endometrial biopsy. It is not unusual to have some irregular bleeding for the first 3 to 6 months on a continuous HRT regimen. Heavy or prolonged bleeding, or any bleeding that occurs after amenorrhea has been established, needs to be evaluated. Bleeding is expected during the pill free interval with cyclic HRT, however prolonged or heavy bleeding requires evaluation (Youngkin & Davis, pp. 418-419; Mishell, p. 1190).

50. **(d)** The benefits of estrogen on bone mass continue for as long as estrogen is taken. Recent evidence suggests that for osteoporosis prevention, estrogen should be continued as long as the woman is ambulatory. Although the benefit is greatest when estrogen is started close to the onset of menopause, it will still slow down bone loss if started several years later. The minimum dosage required for prevention of bone loss is 0.625 mg of conjugated estrogen or the equivalent in other estrogens used for HRT. Transdermal and oral estrogens both have the same beneficial effect on bone (Mishell, pp. 1171-1172).

51. **(a)** By one year postmenopause the ovaries should have become atrophic and should not be palpable. It is recommended that the postmenopausal woman with a palpable ovary be further evaluated (Berek, et al., p. 1166).

52. **(b)** Risk factors identify only 25% of women who will eventually develop breast cancer. The majority of women who get breast cancer do not have apparent risk factors except for gender and age. Only 5% to 10% of breast

cancer is familial. Early menarche and late menopause are less significant as risk factors than family history. One in eight women in the United States will develop breast cancer in her lifetime (Mishell, pp. 361-362).

53. **(d)** The arms are raised above the head during inspection of the breasts to emphasize any changes in the shape or contour of the breasts (Bates, p. 322).

54. **(b)** The American Cancer Society recommendations are for women to begin annual mammography at age 40 (DHHS, p. 259).

55. **(a)** The main function of breast ultrasound is to differentiate between a solid and cystic mass. It may also be useful in the differential diagnosis of masses in the dense breast tissue of younger women (Mishell, pp. 359, 370-371).

56. **(c)** The characteristics of nipple discharge caused by hyperprolactinemia are that it occurs in both breasts, involves multiple ducts, is spontaneous, and is milky and thin in consistency (Arnold & Neiheisel, p. 108).

57. **(b)** Tricyclic antidepressants are one of the many drugs that can cause hyperprolactinemia. Other medications include phenothiazine, metoclopramide, other antidepressants, and several antihypertensives (Arnold & Neiheisel, pp. 106-107).

58. **(d)** The most common cause of spontaneous serous or bloody nipple discharge from a single duct is an intraductal papilloma. Of course, a malignancy must always be considered. The discharge associated with duct ectasia is most often multicolored and sticky. There is no nipple discharge associated with fat necrosis or fibroadenomas (Mishell, pp. 360-361).

59. **(b)** Fibroadenomas are the second most common benign tumor of the breast. They are most common in adolescents and women in their 20s. They are usually single and are firm or rubbery, nontender, and mobile. They do not change in size with the menstrual cycle. Fibrocystic changes are the most common of the benign breast conditions. Symptoms of fibrocystic changes include breast tenderness that is cyclic and often bilateral. Nodularity is a common physical finding. This condition is most common between the ages of 20 and 50. A galactocele is a discrete, milk filled, cystic or firm

mass in the breast of a lactating or recently lactating woman (Mishell, pp. 357-359; Youngkin & Davis, p. 382).

60. **(b)** A modified radical mastectomy is the removal of the entire breast and a sample of lymph nodes, sparing the pectoral muscles. Choice ''a'' describes a radical mastectomy. Choice ''c'' describes a segmental resection (quadrectomy). Choice ''d'' describes a lumpectomy (tylectomy). The modified radical mastectomy and lumpectomy are the two most common surgical approaches for the treatment of breast cancer (Lowdermilk, et al., p. 1251).

61. **(c)** The use of tamoxifen does increase a woman's risk for endometrial cancer. This risk is more than counterbalanced by the decreased risk for recurrence of breast cancer. Tamoxifen is an antiestrogen used as follow-up treatment for women over 50 years old with breast cancers that have estrogen-positive receptors. Women should continue the medication for at least five years. Side effects include hot flashes, nausea and vomiting, fluid retention, weight gain, and thrombocytopenia (Lowdermilk, et al., p. 1253).

62. **(b)** Mifepristone (RU486) acts as an antagonist to block the effect of progesterone. It is 95% effective when used in combination with the prostaglandin misoprostol in the first nine weeks of pregnancy. Misoprostol works by causing uterine contractions to help expel the uterine contents. No serious adverse reactions have been reported with the use of mifepristone or misoprostol (Youngkin & Davis, pp. 212-213).

63. **(d)** The symptoms and the physical examination findings in this situation are indicative of postabortal endometritis. Typical findings with postabortal endometritis not related to retained products of conception include a tender but firm uterus, a closed cervical os with no tissue, and a fever of less than 102° F. With retained products of conception, infection is usually also present. The uterus, however, will be tender, boggy, and enlarged with an open cervical os and possible tissue present. Fever may be greater than 102° F. With a continuing pregnancy, the uterus would be enlarged and nontender, the cervical os would be closed, and there would not be any heavy bleeding or fever. The client would have continuing symptoms of pregnancy. Postabortion syndrome is the result of uterine atony. In this syndrome of unknown cause, the uterus becomes filled with blood in the first few hours after an abortion. The client may have severe pain. The uterus will be

tender, enlarged and boggy. There is minimal vaginal bleeding (Rosenfeld, et al., pp. 326-327).

64. **(d)** The physical changes of aging may have an impact on a woman's sexuality in the following ways: Vaginal lubrication may become less in volume, stimulation may take a longer period of time to occur, orgasms may be shorter, and orgasmic contractions may decrease in strength. Most women do not have a change in level of sexual desire/libido related to the physical changes of aging. Sexual desire seems to be more affected by overall health status, former sexual activity, and partner availability. Some women have an increased sexual interest with age (Youngkin & Davis, p. 407; Rosenfeld, et al., p. 793).

65. **(d)** It is important to obtain and document information concerning activities after the sexual assault such as bathing, changing clothes, and using mouthwash, as these activities may affect the presence of evidence. The total number of partners the victim has ever had is irrelevant to treatment or the collection of evidence, and may be used against the woman if she goes to trial. Questions about more recent sexual activity are appropriate. It is not unusual for emotional status to change quickly from crying to being calm and controlled. Emotional status should be assessed, but judgments as to appropriateness of emotional behavior should not be included in documentation. Rape and sexual assault are legal terms that should not be used in medical documentation unless quoting the victim. It is not the role of the health care provider to prove whether or not a rape occurred (Youngkin & Davis, pp. 874-875; Lowdermilk, et al., pp. 1236-1237).

66. **(c)** Urine or blood toxicology screening for drugs/alcohol is generally not advised as part of the sexual assault assessment unless necessary in providing care for the woman. This information may be used against the victim if she goes to trial. Baseline testing for STDs (including HIV), and for pregnancy if no contraception is being used, are usually performed as part of sexual assault assessment. Of course, none of these tests should be performed without the woman's informed consent (Lowdermilk, et al., p. 1236; Youngkin & Davis, p. 875).

67. **(a)** Women who were exposed in utero to DES are at an increased risk for cervical and vaginal clear cell adenocarcinoma, vaginal adenosis, and

structural abnormalities of the cervix and upper vagina. Colposcopic examination of the vagina and cervix is performed to allow for detailed assessment of the cervicovaginal epithelium. In addition, Pap smears should include specimens from both the cervix and all four quadrants of the vaginal fornices (Mishell, pp. 389-392).

68. **(c)** Toxic shock syndrome (TSS) is caused by absorption of toxins produced by colonized *Staphylococcus aureus*. It is rare but may be fatal and occurs most frequently in menstruating women. Clinical presentation includes fever of 102° F or greater, hypotension, diffuse macular erythema resembling a sunburn, and desquamation of the skin on fingers, toes, palms and soles. Vomiting and diarrhea are often present at the onset of illness. Other signs and symptoms may include severe myalgia, headache, sore throat, and disorientation (Youngkin & Davis, pp. 150-151).

69. **(a)** Colposcopic examination is recommended in some situations even if the Pap smear is normal. These situations include the presence of cervical leukoplakia (white lesions visible to the naked eye), persistent cervical bleeding, and as part of the baseline examination for the HIV positive woman (Hatcher, et al., p. 58).

70. **(b)** Intermenstrual bleeding and postcoital spotting are often the presenting symptoms of endocervical polyps. These polyps occur most frequently in multiparous women in their 40s and 50s. The majority of polyps are benign. Dyspareunia is not a common presenting symptom (Mishell, pp. 479-480)

71. **(b)** The order of the choices in a normal menstrual cycle would be LH surge, ovulation, corpus luteum formation, and peak in progesterone level (Mishell, pp. 101-103; Hatcher, et al., p. 73).

72. **(d)** The endometrial phases in the menstrual cycle include the proliferative phase corresponding with the follicular ovarian phase, the secretory phase corresponding with the luteal ovarian phase and the menstrual phase (Lowdermilk, et al., p. 67; Hatcher, et al., pp. 71-73).

73. **(c)** Near ovulation the cervix feels higher or deeper in the vagina and is soft,

open, and wet. BBT should remain elevated at least 0.4 ° F above the baseline for three days to mark the end of the fertile period. When using the calendar method, the first day of fertility is calculated by subtracting 18 days from the length of the shortest cycle, and the last day of fertility is calculated by subtracting 11 days from the longest cycle. For this couple that would be days 8 through 17 of each menstrual cycle. Before ovulation, the only days that are considered safe are the dry days after menses. The couple should not have unprotected intercourse once they note onset of sticky mucus until the evening of the fourth day after peak mucus day. Peak mucus day is the last day of the clear, slippery spinnbarkeit type mucus (Youngkin & Davis, pp. 203-205).

74. **(c)** The ovum maintains the potential for fertilization for up to 24 hours. Sperm remain viable for about 72 hours (Youngkin & Davis, p. 203; Hatcher, et al., p. 74).

75. **(a)** An appropriately sized diaphragm should not be too tightly pressed against the pubic arch, but allow for one finger tip to fit between the inside of the pubic arch and the anterior edge of the diaphragm. The largest size that is comfortable should be used as vaginal depth increases during sexual arousal and a too small diaphragm may not stay in place. The diaphragm should fit snugly but without tension against the vaginal walls (Hatcher, et al., pp. 397-399).

76. **(b)** The flat spring diaphragm has gentle spring strength and is suitable for the woman who has firm vaginal muscle tone. It may also provide a better fit for the woman who has a shallow notch behind the pubic bone. An arcing spring diaphragm may provide a better fit for the woman with a cystocele, rectocele, or retroverted uterus (Speroff & Darney, p. 235; Hatcher, et al., pp. 390-391).

77. **(b)** The diaphragm should be left in place for at least six hours after the last sexual intercourse as sperm can survive for a few hours in the vagina. The diaphragm should not be left in place longer than 24 hours because of the potential risk for TSS. She should, of course, have used an additional applicator full of spermicide in the vagina before the second and third time she had sexual intercourse (Speroff & Darney, p. 237; Hatcher, et al., pp. 397-399).

78. **(c)** The first dose of hormonal postcoital contraception using oral contraceptive pills should be taken as soon as possible after unprotected sexual intercourse and no later than 72 hours. Effectiveness of the method decreases after this amount of time. Use of hormonal postcoital contraception can, however, still be considered for the woman who presents shortly after 72 hours as this may still reduce the risk of pregnancy and is not likely to be harmful (Speroff & Darney, p. 125; Hatcher, et al., pp. 287-289).

79 **(c)** The second dose of oral contraceptive pills taken as emergency hormonal contraception should be taken 12 hours after taking the first dose (Speroff & Darney, p. 123; Hatcher, et al., p. 278).

80. **(d)** The lactational amenorrhea method has a 1% to 2% failure rate as contraception, for up to six months postpartum, in the breast feeding woman who is amenorrheic and who is not supplementing feedings. To be effective, the infant must be fed on demand without bottle-feeding supplements and only minimal cup or spoon-feeding supplements. Another method of contraception should be initiated when the woman resumes menstruation, decreases breast feeding (e.g., baby sleeping through the night), begins any bottle-feeding, or when the baby turns six months old (Grimes & Wallach, pp. 246-247).

81. **(d)** Progestin only pills have been shown to have no adverse effect on lactation even when started in the first week postpartum. Breast feeding is not a contraindication to the use of combination oral contraceptives. However, their use has been shown to decrease milk supply and may alter the composition of breast milk. If she plans to use combination oral contraceptives with the resumption of menses, they should be started after her first period as ovulation may occur even when periods are irregular (Grimes & Wallach, pp. 248-249).

82. **(b)** There is no firm pharmaceutical evidence that antibiotics decrease the effectiveness of oral contraceptives. If broad spectrum antibiotics have any effect on the bioavailability of estrogen, it is probably only in the first two weeks. This assumption is based on the fact that after two weeks enteric bacteria necessary for enterohepatic recirculation become resistant to the antibiotic. Recommendations in *Contraceptive Technology* (17th ed.), are to use a backup method with antibiotics for the entire duration of treatment or 14 days, whichever is shorter plus another seven days. An increase in the

amount of estrogen is not warranted. There would be no benefit in this situation to change to pills with higher androgenic activity. See the answer rationale for question 83 this section for more information on the androgenic activity of pills and acne. Oral contraceptives do not decrease the effectiveness of antibiotics (Hatcher, et al., pp. 449, 457).

83. **(c)** Recent studies suggest that all oral contraceptives tend to improve acne by suppressing endogenous androgen production. This effect comes from the above described decrease in free testosterone and increase in sex hormone binding globulin levels. Therefore it is unlikely that the client's pill use is causing her acne. There is also no indication that discontinuing her pills while on isotretinoin would result in an exacerbation of her acne. Isotretinoin is a known teratogen. Use in pregnancy has resulted in the birth of infants with severe neurological defects. Oral contraceptives or one of the other highly reliable contraceptive methods should be used while taking isotretinoin (Grimes & Wallach, pp. 51-54, 207; Hatcher, et al., p. 411).

84. **(a)** When levonorgestrel is inserted within the first seven days of the menstrual cycle, it becomes effective immediately. Even if inserted more than seven days after the first day of a period, levonorgestrel levels are high enough within 24 hours of insertion to prevent conception (Grimes & Wallach, p. 132; Speroff & Darney, p. 131).

85. **(a)** It is not unusual for the client to have bruising around the implants after insertion. It is helpful to keep the pressure dressing on for 24 hours after insertion. The bruise usually resolves in 7 to 10 days (Speroff & Darney, p. 151; Hatcher, et al., p. 492).

86. **(c)** It is important to perform a careful bimanual examination prior to IUD insertion. Undetected posterior uterine position is the most common reason for perforation at the time of insertion. The other answer choices would then be performed in the following order; clean the cervix with antiseptic, apply a tenaculum, and sound the uterus (Speroff & Darney, pp. 212, 214-216; Hatcher, et al., p. 524).

87. **(d)** The greatest risk for pelvic infection related to the IUD is at the time of insertion. The relative risk of infection in the first 20 days after insertion is 6.36. The relative risk greater than 20 days after insertion is 1.00. Infection rate may actually be higher when the IUD is inserted during menses. No

consensus has been reached on whether prophylactic antibiotics decrease the incidence of infection. The uterine cavity is sterile again in a short period of time after IUD insertion (Jones, et al., pp. 38-40; Hatcher, et al., p. 522).

88. **(b)** There is an increased risk for preterm labor to occur if the IUD is left in place during pregnancy. There is not an indication for C-section delivery and no risk for congenital anomalies related to the copper in the IUD. IUD removal, when the string is visible, is not associated with an increased risk of spontaneous abortion. There is an increased risk of spontaneous abortion if the IUD is not removed (possibly a septic abortion) or if removal is attempted when the string has drawn up into the uterus (Berek, et al., p. 240; Jones, et al., p. 28).

89. **(b)** Medroxyprogesterone acetate effectiveness is not decreased by the concomitant use of phenytoin or other anti-seizure medications. Actually, medroxyprogesterone acetate has been shown to decrease seizure activity probably due to the sedative properties of progestin. Most of the anti-seizure medications (except sodium valproate) are liver enzyme inducers that cause breakdown of estrogen or progestin. These medications can significantly decrease the effectiveness of levonorgestrel, combination oral contraceptives, and progestin-only pills (Speroff & Darney, pp. 88-89, 123, 137, 177; Hatcher, et al., pp. 474, 478-479).

90. **(d)** According to the 1996 U.S. Collaborative Review of Sterilization (CREST) report, the characteristic most often associated with poststerilization regret in women is younger age at the time of the procedure. Women under 30 were twice as likely to regret their decision as women over 30 at the time of sterilization (Peterson, p. 10; Hatcher, et al., p. 568).

91. **(d)** Usually about 20 ejaculations are required for existing sperm in the vas deferens to be cleared. To be certain of sterility, the man should have a sperm count after having had 20 ejaculations (Mishell, p. 347; Hatcher, et al., p. 581).

92. **(d)** If a woman misses pills in the third week of her pill pack she should finish the rest of the hormonal pills in her pack. She should not take the usual seven days off of hormonal pills but should start a new pack as soon as she finishes that third week of her current pack. In addition, she should use

a backup method until she has taken seven consecutive pills (Hatcher, et al., p. 453).

93. **(c)** The fact that this teenager has been taking oral contraceptives for one year without spotting, and now is having a problem, should alert the clinician that something other than pills may be the cause. Especially with teenagers, the possibility of chlamydia should be considered (Grimes & Wallach, p. 84; Hatcher, et al., p. 439).

94. **(c)** The female condom is made of polyurethane which is stronger than latex. It is intended for one time use. Use along with a male condom is not recommended. Female condoms are more expensive than male latex condoms (Grimes & Wallach, pp. 165-166; Hatcher, et al., pp. 372-374).

95. **(d)** Medroxyprogesterone acetate injections should always be given deep IM to assure optimal effectiveness. In an obese client, the deltoid muscle might be better than the gluteal muscle to assure that administration is deep IM. Massaging the area after injection may lower effectiveness. The dosage is 150 mg and the timing is every three months regardless of a woman's weight (Grimes & Wallach, p. 120; Hatcher, et al., p. 485).

96. **(a)** Ovulation is not always suppressed with progestin-only pills even when they are taken at the same time each day. One of the other main mechanisms of action of progestin-only pills is thickening and decreasing the amount of cervical mucus, making sperm penetration more difficult. This mechanism of action requires that pills be taken very regularly. Cervical mucus may not maintain this quality if pills are taken as little as three hours late, but will return within 48 hours of taking the late pill (Speroff & Darney, pp. 120-121; Hatcher, et al., p. 505).

97. **(c)** It is generally accepted that there is a one week grace period if late receiving DMPA. For consistency in administration practices, the manufacturer's labeling states if the interval between injections is greater than 13 weeks the clinician should determine that the client is not pregnant before administering the next injection. If a sensitive pregnancy test is negative she can receive an injection that day. Asking her to return in one month if she has no menses is not necessary, as she may very likely not have periods (Grimes & Wallach, p. 119; Hatcher, et al., pp. 467, 485-486).

98. **(b)** The rolled rim of the condom should be on the outside. The condom should not be unrolled before it is placed on the penis. The penis should be removed from the vagina while it is still erect and when completely away from her genitals, the condom should be removed. Condoms that are stored properly can be used up to five years past the manufacture date. Latex condoms with spermicide should probably be used within two years of the manufacture date (Speroff & Darney, pp. 254-255; Hatcher, et al., pp. 347-349).

99. **(a)** A contraceptive method such as the diaphragm requires that the user follow instructions correctly each time she has sexual intercourse. This is the reason that the typical failure rate (18%) for the diaphragm is significantly different than the perfect user failure (6%) rate. The IUD, levonorgestrel and tubal sterilization's effectiveness do not depend on having to follow instructions correctly with each intercourse. Typical and perfect use failure rates are the same or less than 1% different with these three methods (Youngkin & Davis, 169; Hatcher, et al., p. 216).

100. **(d)** Oral contraceptive use has been shown to decrease the risk for both ovarian and endometrial cancer (Grimes & Wallach, p. 2-4; Hatcher, et al., p. 410).

101. **(c)** Normal semen analysis characteristics include a total sperm count > 20 million/mL, motility of > 40% with forward progression, morphology > 50% normal, and viability > 60%. Seminal fluid should have a normal viscosity and appearance and a WBC count < 1 million/mL (Hatcher, et al., p. 670).

102. **(b)** This procedure, in addition to being used for evaluation of tubal patency, is in some cases also therapeutic. Post-procedure pregnancy rates are highest when an oil based medium is used. HSG is performed ideally 2 to 5 days after the cessation of menses. This timing reduces risk for infection as well as risk of irradiating an existing pregnancy. In the procedure, radiopaque dye is injected via a cannula through the cervix. Two radiographic views are usually taken, one to demonstrate filling of the uterine cavity and the second at the completion of the procedure to show tubal findings (Berek, pp. 925-926).

103. **(a)** A varicocele is a dilatation of the internal spermatic vein. It is believed to

cause infertility by raising the testicular temperature which causes decreased sperm production (Youngkin & Davis, p. 251).

104. **(a)** Cervical mucus becomes clear, watery, and stretchy, resembling raw egg whites, under the influence of estrogen just prior to ovulation. When allowed to dry, it produces a fern pattern (Youngkin & Davis, p. 205).

105. **(a)** The postcoital test is used to assess the quality of cervical mucus, presence and number of motile sperm in the female reproductive tract after coitus, and the interaction between cervical mucus and sperm. It is recommended that the couple abstain from intercourse for two days prior to the postcoital test. The woman should come into the office for the test within 24 hours after intercourse (ideally within 2 to 12 hours). The test should be performed 1 to 2 days before the anticipated time of ovulation. 48 hours after a positive LH test may be too late, and a rise in BBT indicates that ovulation has occurred (Berek, et al., pp. 925-926).

106. **(b)** Clomiphene citrate is a weak synthetic estrogen that acts as an estrogen agonist for ovulation induction. It blocks estrogen receptors so that the normal ovarian-hypothalamic-estrogen feedback loop is altered. There is then an increase in GnRH release resulting in an increase in gonadotropin secretion. Bromocriptine is an example of a dopamine receptor agonist that may be used in cases of hyperprolactinemia. Human menopausal gonadotropins (hMG), such as menotropins, stimulate follicular development. Treatment with hCG is usually included with hMG to promote oocyte maturation, induce ovulation and maintain the corpus luteum. Pulsatile GnRH administration may be used if the woman has hypothalamic failure (Berek, et al., pp. 936-940).

107. **(b)** Pregnancy rates following a vasectomy reversal are generally 50% or greater. Success depends on the skill of the surgeon, the length of time since the vasectomy was performed, the presence of antisperm antibodies, the age of the female, and the location and length of the vas segment removed. Without testing, there would be no way to know about the presence of antisperm antibodies and there is no known increased risk of birth defects. Studies have indicated that until age 64 a man's age does not affect sperm or the ability to fertilize eggs (Hatcher, et al., pp. 577-578, 658).

108. **(c)** Secondary infertility exists when a couple has previously conceived but is subsequently unable to conceive within 12 months despite having unprotected intercourse. Primary infertility exists when a couple has never conceived despite having unprotected intercourse for at least 12 months. Pregnancy wastage is the term used to describe infertility in which the woman is able to conceive but unable to produce a live birth (Hatcher, et al., p. 654).

109. **(a)** Chlamydia, gonorrhea, trichomoniasis, and herpes cervicitis may all present with vaginal discharge, dysuria, postcoital bleeding, and cervical friability. The wet mount will demonstrate many WBCs. The differentiating piece of information is that gonorrhea is the only one of these infections caused by gram negative diplococcus (Youngkin & Davis, pp. 275-278).

110. **(a)** One of the CDC recommended treatment regimens for uncomplicated gonorrhea in a nonpregnant female is ceftriaxone 125 mg IM in a single dose plus doxycycline 100 mg orally twice a day for seven days (CDC, p. 61).

111. **(d)** Molluscum contagiosum is caused by a virus. Lesions are typically dome-shaped, waxy papules with central umbilications. They are usually 1 to 5 mm in size, flesh to white colored, and occur most commonly on the trunk and anogenital region. They are not painful or pruritic. The lesions of acne vulgaris include open and closed comedones, inflammatory papules and pustules. Erythema nodosum presents as very tender lesions that are pink or red and are 1 to 10 cm in diameter. Folliculitis is an inflammatory reaction in a hair follicle characterized by a pustular lesion with central hair (Lommel, et al., pp. 262, 278).

112. **(a)** Molluscum contagiosum is a self-limiting infection often resolving spontaneously within a few months. If the infection is bothersome, cryotherapy with liquid nitrogen may be used for destruction of lesions. If there are only a few lesions they can be unroofed with a sterile needle to remove the central core (Youngkin & Davis, p. 294).

113. **(b)** Systemic symptoms such as malaise and low-grade fever may occur with a primary or initial herpes episode. Such symptoms are less likely with recurrent episodes. The risk of herpes transmission exists both during asymptomatic periods and when there are prodromal symptoms. Topical therapy with acyclovir is less effective than oral therapy. Treatment of recurrent herpes

episodes during pregnancy with any of the antivirals is not recommended (Hatcher, et al., pp. 195-196; CDC, pp. 21-25).

114. **(b)** A Tzanck preparation is obtained from a scraping of the suspect lesion. Multinucleated giant cells with intranuclear inclusions are seen with herpes simplex (Hatcher, et al., p. 195).

115. **(d)** The Jarisch-Herxheimer reaction is an acute febrile reaction with headache and myalgia that may occur within 24 hours after any therapy for syphilis. It occurs most commonly in individuals with early syphilis. Antipyretics may be recommended for symptomatic relief. It is not an allergic reaction to medication. There is no proven method to prevent this adverse reaction (CDC, p. 30).

116. **(c)** The RPR (and VDRL) are nontreponemal tests. It is expected that these tests will eventually become nonreactive after treatment. The FTA-ABs (and MHA-TP) are both treponemal tests. Most individuals who have had syphilis will have a positive treponemal test for the remainder of their lives. There are exceptions for both of the above but they are just that—exceptions rather than the normal expected findings (CDC, p. 29).

117. **(c)** According to the CDC, empiric treatment of PID should be initiated in sexually active young women and others at risk for STDs if the following minimum criteria are present and no other cause for the illness can be identified; lower abdominal tenderness, adnexal tenderness, and cervical motion tenderness (CDC, p. 80).

118. **(b)** A positive Darkfield examination of lesion exudate is diagnostic of primary syphilis. The CDC recommended treatment for primary syphilis is benzathine penicillin G 2.4 million units IM in a single dose (CDC, pp. 29, 31).

119. **(a)** Vaginal candidiasis presents with vaginal itching and discharge, dyspareunia, vulvar dysuria, and vaginal burning, irritation and soreness. Symptoms will frequently increase just prior to menses. Diagnostic findings include a normal pH, negative amine, and a wet mount showing no clue cells, few

WBCs, and the presence of hyphae, pseudohyphae, buds or filaments. Treatment will be with an antifungal agent such as terconazole. In bacterial vaginosis, the pH is > 4.5, amine is negative, and a wet mount will demonstrate clue cells. Trichomoniasis will demonstrate a pH > 5, many WBCs, and possibly motile trichomonads (CDC, pp. 75-76).

120. **(c)** The currently available treatments for genital warts do not eradicate the virus. The CDC currently recommends that treatment of partners is not necessary for the management of genital warts. Annual Pap smears are recommended unless there is a Pap smear abnormality. If genital warts are located on the cervix, a Pap smear should be done to assess for high grade squamous intraepithelial lesions prior to treatment (CDC, pp. 88, 92-93).

121. **(a)** *Haemophilus ducreyi* is the causative organism in chancroid. The appearance of a painful genital ulcer and tender inguinal lymphadenopathy suggests a diagnosis of chancroid. When the above findings are accompanied by a suppurative inguinal adenopathy (bubo) the diagnosis of chancroid is almost certain (CDC, p. 19).

122. **(d)** Trichomoniasis usually presents with a foul smelling vaginal discharge and itching. Dysuria and dyspareunia may also be present. Examination findings include presence of a frothy, yellow-green vaginal discharge and vulvar erythema. Petechial lesions may also be seen on the cervix and are sometimes called strawberry marks. Male partners are usually asymptomatic, but may have symptoms of urethritis or prostatitis (Youngkin & Davis, p. 274).

References

Arnold, G., & Neiheisel, M. (1997). A comprehensive approach to evaluating nipple discharge. *The Nurse Practitioner: The American Journal of Primary Health Care, 22*(7), 96-111.

Bates, B. (1995). *A guide to physical examination and history taking* (6th ed.). Philadelphia: J. B. Lippincott.

Berek, J., Adashi, E. Y., & Hillard, P. (Eds.). (1996). *Novak's gynecology* (12th ed.). Baltimore: Williams & Wilkins.

Blackwell, R. (1996). *Women's medicine.* Cambridge, MA: Blackwell Science, Inc.

Brinton, L. (1996). Cigarette smoking and endometrial, ovarian and cervical cancers. *Association of Reproductive Health Practitioners Clinical Proceedings*, October, 8-10.

Centers for Disease Control and Prevention (CDC). (1998). 1998 Guidelines for treatment of sexually transmitted diseases. *MMWR* 47 (No. RR-1).

Dains, J., Baumann, L., & Scheibel, P. (1998). *Advanced health assessment and clinical diagnosis in primary care.* St. Louis: Mosby.

Department of Health and Human Services (DHHS). (1998). *Clinician's handbook of preventive services* (2nd ed.). Washington, DC: U.S. Government Printing Office.

Grimes, D., & Wallach, M. (1997). *Modern contraception: Updates from the contraception report.* Totowa, NJ: Emron.

Hatcher, R., Trussell, J., Stewart, F., Cates, W., Stewart, G. K., Guest, F., & Kowal, D. (1998). *Contraceptive technology* (17th ed.). New York: Ardent Media.

Havens, C., Sullivan, N., & Tilton, P. (1996). *Manual of outpatient gynecology* (3rd ed.). Boston: Little, Brown, & Co.

Jones, H., Jaffe, R., Cefalo, R., & Bowes, W. (1996). IUDS: A state of the art conference. *Supplement to: Obstetrical and Gynecological Survey, 51*(12).

Krummel. D., & Kris-Etherton, P. (1996). *Nutrition in women's health.* Gaithersburg, MD: Aspen Publishers.

Lommel, L., & Jackson, P. (1997). *Assessing and managing common signs and symptoms.* San Francisco: University of California San Francisco Nursing Press.

Lowdermilk. D., Perry, S., & Bobak, I. (1997). *Maternity and women's health care* (6th ed.). St. Louis: Mosby.

Mashburn, J., & Scharbo-DeHaan, M. (1997). A clinician's guide to pap smear interpretation. *The Nurse Practitioner: The American Journal of Primary Health Care, 22*(4), 115-143.

Millonig, V. (1996). *Today and tomorrow's woman: Menopause: Before and after.* Potomac, MD: Health Leadership Associates.

Mishell, D., Stenchever, M., Droegemueller, W., & Herbst, A. (1997). *Comprehensive gynecolgy* (3rd ed.). St. Louis: Mosby.

Murphy, J. (Ed.). (1998). Raloxifene. *Nurse practitioners' prescribing reference, 5*(2), 186.

Peterson, H. (1996). Update on female sterilization: Failure rates, counseling issues, and post-sterilization regret. *The Contraception Report, 7*(3), 4-11.

Rosenfeld, J. (1997). *Women's health in primary care.* Baltimore: Williams & Wilkins.

Speroff, L., & Darney, P. (1996) *A clinical guide for contraception* (2nd ed.). Baltimore: Williams & Wilkins.

Youngkin, E., & Davis, M. (1998). *Women's health: A primary care clinical guide* (2nd ed.). Stamford, CT: Appleton & Lange.

Obstetrics

Beth Kelsey
Anne Salomone

Select one best answer to the following questions.

1. A common discomfort in pregnancy that may occur as a result of increased progesterone levels is:

   a. Constipation
   b. Gum bleeding
   c. Low back pain
   d. Nasal stuffiness

2. A pregnant woman is 5'6" in height has a prepregnant weight of 130 lbs. Which of the following would represent the most appropriate weight for her by the end of her pregnancy?

   a. 145 lbs
   b. 150 lbs
   c. 165 lbs
   d. 170 lbs

3. A client presents for her first prenatal visit. She does not remember exactly when her last normal period was, and has been taking oral contraceptives until yesterday when she found out she was pregnant. She denies feeling any fetal movement. Fundal height is half way between the symphysis and umbilicus. Your initial assessment of her gestation given this information is that she is:

   a. 12 weeks pregnant
   b. 16 weeks pregnant
   c. 20 weeks pregnant
   d. 24 weeks pregnant

4. Relief from heartburn during pregnancy may be obtained by:

    a. Drinking a large glass of water with meals
    b. Eating 5 or 6 small meals each day
    c. Lying down for 30 minutes after meals
    d. Taking an antacid such as sodium bicarbonate

5. A woman presents with the complaints of no menses for three months, nausea, breast tenderness, and urinary frequency. She believes she is pregnant. These signs are classified as:

    a. Presumptive signs of pregnancy
    b. Probable signs of pregnancy
    c. Positive signs of pregnancy
    d. Objective signs of pregnancy

6. Upon auscultating the heart of a pregnant woman who is 16-weeks-gestation you notice that she has a split S_1. Appropriate management would include:

    a. Advising her to limit her physical activity
    b. Re-evaluating her heart in the third trimester
    c. Recognizing that this is a normal finding
    d. Scheduling an echocardiogram

7. A woman is currently 12-weeks-pregnant and has had three full term deliveries. One of these babies died at four months from SIDS. She has also had one stillbirth at 34 weeks and one spontaneous abortion. Which of the following correctly represents her pregnancy history?

    a. Gravida (G) 5, Term (T) 4, Preterm (P) 0, Abortion (A) 1, Living (L) 3
    b. G5 T3 P1 A1 L2
    c. G6 T3 P0 A2 L3
    d. G6 T3 P1 A1 L2

8. Human chorionic gonadotropin (hCG) is produced by the:

    a. Corpus luteum
    b. Pituitary gland
    c. Placenta
    d. Trophoblast

9. Which thyroid hormone remains within nonpregnant normal limits during pregnancy?

a. TSH
b. Total T_4
c. TBG
d. Total T_3

10. Using Nägele's rule, the estimated date of delivery (EDD) for a pregnant woman with a LMP of November 20 would be:

    a. August 6
    b. August 13
    c. August 20
    d. August 27

11. A PPD test is done as part of routine screening for a 12-weeks-pregnant client who has no risk factors for tuberculosis. The test is positive with an induration of 15 mm. Management for this client should include:

    a. Obtaining a chest radiograph after delivery
    b. Obtaining a chest radiograph now
    c. Immediate initiation of isoniazid
    d. Initiation of isoniazid after delivery

12. Current ACOG guidelines, based on CDC recommendations, are that all pregnant women be tested for HIV infection. In counseling the pregnant client prior to testing you would advise her that if she is infected with HIV:

    a. Cesarean section delivery is recommended to decrease the chance of the infant becoming infected at the time of birth
    b. Labor will likely be induced at 38 weeks to reduce the length of time that the infant is exposed to the virus
    c. She can be given medication after the first trimester to reduce the risk of the infant becoming infected
    d. Termination of the pregnancy is recommended as most HIV infected infants die within the first three years after birth

13. A 27-year-old G2 P0 Mediterranean female presents for a routine visit at 27-weeks-gestation. She relates that she has discontinued taking her prenatal vitamins as she believes they are making the skin around her eyes and face darken. You advise her that:

    a. She should change to a supplement that does not contain iron
    b. This may be due to a hereditary type of anemia
    c. Getting some sun exposure will help to even out the color

    d. The darker pigmentation usually fades after the baby is born

14. The hormone chorionic somatomammotropin (or human placental lactogen or hPL):

    a. Stimulates the growth of the breasts and has lactogenic properties
    b. Causes a relaxation of the joints resulting in the 'waddle' of pregnancy
    c. Promotes the development of oxytocin receptors in the cervix
    d. Causes vasodilation and the drop in blood pressure seen in the second trimester

15. Expected pelvic examination findings at eight weeks gestation include:

    a. Braxton Hicks contractions
    b. Dextrorotation of the uterus
    c. Softening of the uterine isthmus
    d. Uterus palpable at the symphysis pubis

16. The hormone relaxin is responsible for the:

    a. Let-down reflex
    b. Onset of labor
    c. Dilatation of the ureters
    d. Softening of pelvic ligaments

17. Hemodynamic changes that occur during pregnancy include:

    a. Decrease in heart rate and increase in systemic vascular resistance
    b. Decrease in systemic vascular resistance and increase in cardiac output
    c. Increase in heart rate and increase in systemic vascular resistance
    d. Increase in systemic vascular resistance and decrease in cardiac output

18. Results of a urine culture from a clean catch urine specimen obtained at an initial prenatal visit indicate the presence of 50,000 *E. coli* per mL of urine. The client currently has no urinary complaints. Appropriate management would include:

    a. Instructing the client that no treatment is needed at this time but to report any urinary tract infection symptoms
    b. Repeating the urine culture to assure that the results were not due to contamination
    c. Initiating antibiotic therapy and repeating the urine culture two weeks after treatment is completed

d. Initiating suppressive therapy and checking urine at each visit for nitrites or leukocyte esterase

19. A 32-weeks-pregnant client complains of frequent leg cramps. She currently drinks four, eight ounce glasses of milk each day and walks 30 minutes each day for exercise. Interventions to decrease this client's leg cramps would include:

   a. Alternately flexing and extending the feet
   b. Decreasing the amount of daily walking
   c. Taking aluminum hydroxide gel with meals
   d. Taking a daily phosphorus supplement

20. Folic acid supplementation prior to conception has been shown to decrease the incidence of:

   a. Cardiac anomalies
   b. Down syndrome
   c. Neural tube defects
   d. Spontaneous abortion

21. In the pre-embryonic stage, the inner cell mass called the blastocyst will eventually become the:

   a. Yolk sac, amnion, and placenta
   b. Second polar body
   c. Embryo, amnion, and yolk sac membrane
   d. Maternal side of the chorion and placenta

22. The gestational age at greatest risk for taking a drug that can cause cardiac anomalies is:

   a. 1 to 3 weeks
   b. 3 to 7 weeks
   c. 7 to 10 weeks
   d. 10 to 14 weeks

23. The corpus luteum cyst is responsible for secreting:

   a. hCG to maintain the pregnancy during the first trimester
   b. Progesterone to maintain the uterine lining for implantation
   c. Human placental lactogen to promote placental formation
   d. Prolactin to promote growth of the ductal system of the breasts

24. A normal hematological change you would expect to see during pregnancy would include an increase in:

   a. WBC count
   b. Hematocrit
   c. Platelet count
   d. Serum ferritin

25. A 10-weeks-pregnant woman has stepped on a rusty piece of metal requiring several stitches to close the laceration. Her last tetanus injection was 10 years ago. Appropriate advice would include telling her that:

   a. She should not receive the tetanus booster while she is in her first trimester
   b. If she received a complete primary series of three injections a booster is not needed
   c. The tetanus vaccine is a toxoid and is considered safe to give during pregnancy
   d. Tetanus immune globulin should be given rather than a booster vaccination

26. A frantic client calls your office today. She is 28-weeks-pregnant and her husband has just been diagnosed with varicella. She relates that she had chicken pox when she was a teenager, but she has heard that chicken pox is very serious for pregnant women as the baby may still become infected. You advise her that she should:

   a. Receive (varicella zoster immunoglobulin) VZIG
   b. Avoid contact with her husband until he is well again
   c. Have a varicella titer drawn to confirm her immunity
   d. Have a targeted ultrasound to check the fetus for signs of infection

27. Amniocentesis is not able to detect:

   a. Birth defects related to teratogen exposure
   b. Fetal lung maturity
   c. Amnionitis
   d. Fetal hemolytic disease (Rh or anti-D)

28. By definition, a reactive NST demonstrates:

   a. A minimum of two or more accelerations in the fetal heart rate of 10 beats or more, for 10 or more seconds, in a 10 minute period

b. Two or more decelerations in the fetal heart rate of 10 or more beats, for 10 or more seconds, in a 10 minute period

c. A minimum of two or more accelerations in the fetal heart rate of 15 or more beats, for 15 or more seconds, in a 20 minute period

d. A minimum of four or more accelerations in the fetal heart rate of 15 or more beats, for 15 or more seconds, in a 15 minute period

29. During an ultrasound examination, a 32-week-pregnant woman states that she is feeling dizzy and lightheaded. She is diaphoretic and pale. This woman is most likely experiencing:

    a. An anxiety attack
    b. Hypoglycemia
    c. Orthostatic hypotension
    d. Vena cava syndrome

30. The result of a biophysical profile (BPP) performed at 36-weeks-gestation reveals a score of 6 including a normal amniotic fluid volume. Counseling for this client should include that:

    a. The biophysical profile will need to be repeated in one week
    b. She will probably have a contraction stress test scheduled
    c. Nonstress tests will be scheduled twice weekly until delivery
    d. Delivery may be considered at this time if the fetus is mature

31. Instructions on monitoring fetal activity for a pregnant woman who is 32-weeks-gestation should include which of the following?

    a. Expect a noticeable increase in movement as the pregnancy nears term
    b. There should be at least 10 movements identified in a one hour period
    c. Monitor fetal movement daily in the morning After eating breakfast
    d. Vary the time of day for counting to ensure an adequate assessment

32. A 38-weeks-pregnant diabetic client is being evaluated for possible induction of labor because of concerns about macrosomia. In determining the chances for a successful induction, Bishop's scoring is done. The components of this scoring include evaluation for:

    a. Cervical consistency
    b. Loss of the mucous plug
    c. Position of the fetus
    d. Rupture of membranes

Questions 33 and 34 refer to the following monitor strip.

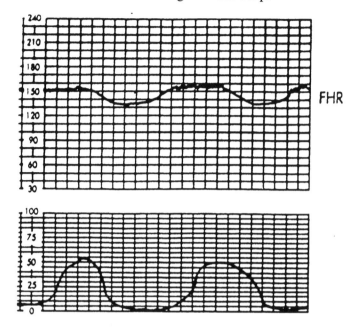

33. The most likely cause of the type of the decelerations seen on the above monitor strip is:

    a. Fetal sleep cycling
    b. Head compression
    c. Umbilical cord compression
    d. Uteroplacental insufficiency

34. A laboring woman, whose only medication has been meperidine hydrochloride 50 mg IM, has the above monitor strip reading. Management for this woman would include:

    a. Administering an opiate antagonist such as naloxone
    b. Continuing routine care and fetal heart rate monitoring
    c. Performing a vaginal examination to assess for a prolapsed cord
    d. Turning her on her left side and administering oxygen

35. A 36-weeks-pregnant client with possible intrauterine growth retardation (IUGR) has a negative contraction stress test. The most likely intervention will be:

    a. Follow-up with a biophysical profile

b. Immediate delivery by C-section
c. Repeating the test in 24 to 48 hours
d. Repeating the test in one week

36. The following is recorded as findings from a vaginal examination of a laboring woman with a fetus in vertex position: 50%, 3 cm, -1. Which of the following would be a correct interpretation of this data?

    a. Dilatation of the cervix is 50% complete
    b. The cervix length is 3 centimeters
    c. The fetal head is above the ischial spines
    d. The fetal presenting part is floating

37. A client presents with a positive urine hCG and LNMP of 8 weeks. She states she has had a small amount of bright red vaginal bleeding for the past 12 hours. She is also having mild abdominal cramping pain. A pelvic examination reveals a closed cervix and a slightly tender uterus with a size that corresponds with her LNMP. The differential diagnosis for this woman includes:

    a. Ectopic pregnancy and inevitable abortion
    b. Ectopic pregnancy and threatened abortion
    c. Implantation bleeding and threatened abortion
    d. Inevitable abortion and incomplete abortion

38. Expected serial quantitative hCG levels for a normal intrauterine pregnancy should double every:

    a. 12 hours
    b. 24 hours
    c. 48 hours
    d. 72 hours

39. The CDC recommended management of condyloma acuminata during pregnancy is:

    a. Application of podophyllin to external condyloma only
    b. Application of trichloroacetic acid to condyloma
    c. Application of imiquimod 5% cream to condyloma
    d. Delay of any treatment until after delivery

40. A 28-year-old woman presents to your office stating she had a positive urine hCG at the health department four months ago. Her urine pregnancy test today

is again positive. Physical examination reveals a normal sized uterus with a normal pelvic examination. Ultrasound in the office reveals no evidence of pregnancy. You realize that:

    a. This is a rare but possible occurrence and have her return in six months to see if the hCG has reverted to negative

    b. There are false positives to all urine pregnancy tests and this is probably one of them

    c. This occurs in any condition where there is a FSH surge, and both times the hCG was measured she may have been ovulating

    d. This may occur in some types of cancer and warrants further evaluation

41. A couple presents for genetic counseling. They are both autosomal recessive for sickle cell anemia. You can tell them that their risk for having an infant born with sickle cell disease is:

    a. 1 in 4 chance (25%)

    b. 2 in 4 chance (50%)

    c. 4 in 4 chance (100%)

    d. No chance (0%)

42. When using ultrasound assessment to determine an EDD, the most accurate dating can be obtained from:

    a. Crown rump length (CRL) at eight weeks gestation

    b. Abdominal circumference at 16 weeks gestation

    c. Biparietal diameter (BPD) at 20 weeks gestation

    d. Femur length (FL) at 30 weeks gestation

43. Which of the following statements concerning chorionic villi sampling is true?

    a. Both chromosomal and DNA information can be obtained

    b. The test is useful in the early diagnosis of neural tube defects

    c. The test is ideally performed prior to 10 weeks gestations

    d. Pregnancy loss rates are higher than with amniocentesis

44. Which of the following pregnant clients would be most at risk for intrauterine growth retardation (IUGR)?

    a. 17 year old, G1 P0 with a Hgb of 11.8 at 30 weeks

    b. 24 year old, G2 P1 with a previous preterm birth

    c. 28 year old, G1 P0 with chronic hypertension

    d. 32 year old, G2 P1 who is 120% of ideal body weight

45. A 26-weeks-pregnant Rh negative client is in an automobile accident and feto-maternal hemorrhage is suspected. Which of the following tests would be used to determine the dose of Rh-immune globulin to be given to this client?

    a. Direct Coombs
    b. Indirect Coombs
    c. Kleihauer-Betke
    d. Rh antibody titer

46. One treatment for ectopic pregnancy is the use of methotrexate. This drug works by:

    a. Stopping the growth of the corpus luteum
    b. Increasing the peristalsis of the fallopian tube
    c. Inhibiting DNA synthesis and cell multiplication
    d. Causing a disruption of the endometrium

47. Which of the following supplements should be avoided during treatment for ectopic pregnancy with methotrexate?

    a. Calcium
    b. Folic acid
    c. Iron
    d. Vitamin B$_{12}$

48. A 28-year-old client is being seen for her initial prenatal visit at 10 weeks gestation. She states she is used to running a distance of five miles 4 to 5 times a week and wants to know if she can continue this exercise routine. The most appropriate response would be to tell this client that:

    a. She should enroll in an aerobics class as there is less risk of muscle injury
    b. She should walk to decrease the risk for fetal hyperthermia
    c. She can continue to run but should decrease the frequency to 2 to 3 times a week
    d. She should monitor her weight gain to assure she is getting adequate calories

Questions 49 and 50 refer to the following scenario.

49. A 40-year-old G1 P0 at 32 weeks gestation presents with bright red vaginal bleeding for the past six hours, back pain, and irregular, abdominal, crampy

pain that she describes as colicky. Her pregnancy has been complicated by chronic hypertension and only a 5 lb weight gain. She smokes two packs of cigarettes per day. Routine ultrasound surveillance has been unremarkable. Examination reveals no CVA tenderness, FHR 120 bpm, no abdominal tenderness, fundal height of 33 cm with increased uterine tone, and the vertex dipping into the pelvis. Vital signs are unchanged from previous visits. Given this information, you suspect:

    a. Marginal placenta previa
    b. Hemorrhagic cystitis
    c. HELLP syndrome
    d. Placental abruption

50. The immediate plan of care for this client in addition to obtaining a CBC and blood type with crossmatch, should include:

    a. Continuous fetal monitoring, urinalysis, and CAT scan of the pelvis
    b. Chemistry profile, 24 hour urine for protein and creatinine clearance, and intermittent fetal monitoring
    c. Ultrasound, intermittent fetal monitoring, and 24 hour urine for protein and creatinine clearance
    d. Ultrasound, continuous fetal monitoring, and coagulation studies

51. Increased risk for placental abruption has been associated with:

    a. Cocaine use
    b. Diabetes
    c. Obesity
    d. Pyelonephritis

52. HELLP syndrome stands for:

    a. Hypertension, elevated leukocytes, low platelets
    b. Hypertension, elevated liver enzymes, lethargy, proteinuria
    c. Hemolysis, elevated liver enzymes, low platelets
    d. Hemolysis, elevated leukocytes, lethargy, proteinuria

53. A client presents with complaints of right upper quadrant pain and headache for 24 hours. Physical examination reveals fundal height consistent with the estimated gestational age of 32 weeks, good fetal movement, 1+ edema of feet, and 1+ proteinuria. Her BP is 136/88 (baseline from first visit 110/65) and pulse is 100. You suspect:

    a. Pyelonephritis

b. Pre-eclampsia
c. Early preterm labor
d. Cholecystitis

54. Risk factors for asymptomatic bacteriuria in pregnancy include:

a. Multiple pregnancy
b. Premature labor
c. Hypertension
d. Sickle cell disease

55. Gestational diabetes results from abnormal glucose metabolism because of the:

a. Insulin antagonist action of hPL, estrogen, and progesterone
b. Insulin antagonist action of the fetal placenta and fetal antibodies
c. Suppression of insulin secretion from the maternal pancreas due to estradiol
d. Increased insulin needs of the mother and fetus during pregnancy

56. The recommended time schedule for gestational diabetes screening is:

a. Whenever the initial prenatal laboratory tests are performed
b. With initial prenatal laboratory tests and at 28 weeks
c. Between 24 and 28 weeks of gestation
d. Each trimester if the woman has diabetes risk factors

57. A diagnosis of gestational diabetes is made when:

a. The one hour plasma value is 150 mg
b. One or more values on plasma samples are exceeded: Fasting—105 mg, 1 hour—190 mg, 2 hour—165 mg, 3 hour—145 mg
c. Two or more values on plasma samples are exceeded: Fasting—105 mg, 1 hour—190 mg, 2 hour—165 mg, 3 hour—145 mg
d. Three or more values on plasma samples are exceeded: Fasting—120 mg, 1 hour—145 mg, 2 hour—130 mg, 3 hour—110 mg

58. A woman with diabetes who would like to become pregnant has come to the office for preconception counseling. She currently takes regular and NPH insulin twice a day. Counseling for this client should include the following information:

a. A glycosylated hemoglobin level should be obtained prior to conception
b. She will need to change to an oral hypoglycemic prior to conception
c. She will probably need to increase her insulin dosage in the first trimester

    d. Strict glucose control prior to conception will prevent fetal macrosomia

59. A pregnant woman who is vegetarian but does eat yogurt and cheese is most likely to be deficient in:

    a. Folic acid
    b. Iron
    c. Protein
    d. Vitamin B_{12}

60. A 39-weeks-pregnant client presents with a mild sore throat and nasal congestion. Her temperature is 99.8° F. Appropriate relief measures would include:

    a. Aspirin and increase fluid intake
    b. Acetaminophen and a nasal decongestant spray
    c. Ibuprofen and salt water gargles
    d. Naproxen and pseudoephedrine

61. An Rh negative pregnant woman should be given Rho (D) immune globulin (RhoGAM) after delivery if she has a:

    a. Negative indirect Coombs test and the baby is Rh negative
    b. Positive indirect Coombs test and the baby is Rh negative
    c. Negative indirect Coombs test and the baby is Rh positive
    d. Positive indirect Coombs test and the baby is Rh positive

62. A blood antibody screen demonstrates a Kell antibody. You know that Kell:

    a. Isoimmunization can occur and can produce erythroblastosis fetalis
    b. Antibodies are associated with a recent viral illness and are insignificant
    c. Is from a prior transfusion and is not significant to the fetus but will make it more difficult to find a crossmatch for the mother
    d. Antibody formation can be prevented by administering RhoGAM

63. There would be a risk for fetal ABO hemolytic disease if a mother who was:

    a. Type A, delivered an infant who was type O
    b. Type B, delivered an infant who was type O
    c. Type O, delivered an infant who was type A
    d. Type AB, delivered an infant who was type O

64. A Liley graph (optical density graph) is used in Rh-sensitized pregnancies to assess the risk to the fetus of an adverse outcome by plotting:

    a. The mother's antibody titers
    b. Amniotic fluid bilirubin levels
    c. Fetal hemoglobin levels
    d. Predictive ultrasound parameters

65. A 25-year-old primiparous woman who is 17-weeks-gestation is being seen to-day for a routine antepartum visit. She is scheduled to have a maternal serum alpha-fetoprotein (MSAFP) drawn at this visit. She now states that she is not sure that she wants this test done because several of her friends had the test come back "abnormal." They worried the whole pregnancy that something was wrong with their babies, but all were born normal. In counseling her, you:

    a. Acknowledge her fear, and explain that false positives only occur if gesta-tional dates are inaccurate
    b. Explain that the MSAFP test is a screening test and only indicates individ-uals who may warrant further testing
    c. Explain that the test is usually repeated in 4 to 8 weeks if the initial re-sults are abnormal
    d. Advise her that she can cancel the test today and reschedule it anytime if she decides that she does want it

66. The most common preventable type of birth defect in the United States is:

    a. Neural tube defects
    b. Fetal alcohol syndrome
    c. Intrauterine growth retardation
    d. Down syndrome

67. A 28-year-old G1 P0 client presents for her first prenatal visit. You find that she has a history of genital herpes and a lesion on her labia minora. She relates she has one to two outbreaks a year. You counsel her that:

    a. Prophylactic therapy with acyclovir is recommended after the first trimes-ter to prevent perinatal transmission
    b. She will need Cesarean delivery to prevent perinatal transmission
    c. She will need to have a careful perineal examination when she presents for delivery and if no lesions are present she can have a vaginal delivery
    d. She will need serial cervical cultures for HSV starting at 32 weeks. If any are positive she will need a Cesarean delivery

68. A woman presents to your office today with a positive pregnancy test. She is at 12 weeks gestation. She relates that she received a rubella vaccine six weeks ago and asks if this is a problem. She should be counseled that:

a. A targeted ultrasound should be considered as it will show if there are any major birth defects
b. Although the vaccine is not recommended in pregnancy there has been no documented evidence that it causes birth defects
c. She received the vaccine after most of the major organs were developed so the risk to the fetus is minimal
d. Termination of pregnancy should be considered due to the serious birth defects caused by rubella

69. TORCH titer stands for:

a. Toxoplasmosis; Oral herpes; Rubella; Chlamydia; genital Herpes
b. Toxoplasmosis; Oral herpes; Rubella; Chlamydia; Hepatitis
c. Toxoplasmosis; Other infections; Rubella; Cytomegalovirus; Herpes
d. Toxoplasmosis; Other infections; Rubella; Cytomegalovirus; Hepatitis

70. A woman is exposed to human parvovirus (fifth disease) during the 24th week of gestation. You know that:

a. Fetal infection is likely and there is a high chance of preterm labor or stillbirth
b. Half of women are immune to fifth disease but if she is not she is likely to contract the illness and preterm labor is likely
c. Half of women are immune to fifth disease, but even with close exposure the highest risk of contracting the disease is 50%
d. The viral load will determine if it is a problem for the fetus

71. Polyhydramnios is associated with:

a. Maternal hypertension
b. Neural tube defects
c. Post-term pregnancy
d. Pulmonary hypoplasia

72. A fetal anomaly that would increase the likelihood of oligohydramnios is:

a. Esophageal atresia
b. Hydrocephalus
c. Renal agenesis
d. Meningomyelocele

73. The diagnosis of ruptured membranes is definitive when:

a. Fluid is seen escaping from the cervical os

b. Nitrazine paper turns blue when placed in the vagina
c. Slide of dried cervical secretions have a fern-like appearance
d. The patient reports a gush of fluid from the vagina

74. You are giving your near term patient instructions on when to go to the hospital. You tell her that true labor contractions should be regular and should be timed from the:

a. Beginning of one contraction to the beginning of the next contraction
b. End of one contraction to the beginning of the next contraction
c. End of one contraction to the end of the next contraction
d. Peak of one contraction to the peak of the next contraction

75. A second degree laceration involves the vaginal mucosa:

a. Posterior fourchette, and perineal skin
b. Posterior fourchette, periurethral area, and perineal skin
c. Posterior fourchette, perineal skin, and perineal muscles
d. Periurethral area, perineal skin, and external anal sphincter

76. First stage of labor is defined as lasting from the onset of:

a. Contractions until active cervical dilatation occurs
b. Regular contractions with cervical change until transition
c. Regular contractions with cervical change until complete dilatation
d. Cervical change until the delivery of the infant

77. During a routine antepartum visit your patient asks what is the usual monitoring procedure for the baby during labor. Since she has no identified risks you advise her that the usual guidelines for monitoring fetal heart rate in labor are:

a. To check the FHR at least every 30 minutes during the first stage of active labor and every 15 minutes during the second stage of labor
b. Continuous fetal monitoring after the cervix has dilated to 8 cm or membranes have ruptured
c. To check the FHR every hour during the first stage of active labor, every 30 minutes during transition and every 15 minutes during the second stage of labor
d. Continuous fetal monitoring whenever the patient is in bed but can be discontinued whenever she wants to get up to walk

78. What is the normal mechanism for labor in a vertex presentation?

   a. Descent, engagement, internal rotation, flexion, external rotation, restitution

   b. Engagement, descent, internal rotation, flexion, restitution, external rotation

   c. Internal rotation, engagement, descent, restitution, flexion, external rotation

   d. Engagement, descent, flexion, internal rotation, restitution, external rotation

79. A 27-year-old G2 P1 had a C-section with her last delivery because of a transverse lie. She relates that they told her that the baby was "stuck" in the top of her uterus and they had to "do a extra little cut up there" to get him out. You note that she has a Pfannenstiel incision on her abdomen. She is interested in having a vaginal birth after Cesarean section (VBAC) with this pregnancy. You tell her that:

   a. She is probably a candidate for a VBAC if the baby is less than 4000 g

   b. She is not a candidate for a VBAC assuming the medical records confirm her story

   c. As long as she does not require pitocin she should be able to have a VBAC

   d. As long as the fetus is not in a transverse lie, she should be able to have a VBAC

80. A 25-year-old G1 P0 at 38 weeks gestation has had an uncomplicated pregnancy. She presents today for a routine visit. She relates that the baby was extremely active yesterday but has not moved today. She states she is having a few contractions and lost her mucus plug four days ago. Given this information you:

   a. Recognize that it is common to have the baby stop moving shortly before labor

   b. Are concerned that there is a problem because of the lack of fetal movement

   c. Recognize that labor is imminent as she has lost her mucous plug

   d. Do a sterile speculum examination to check for ruptured membranes

81. In a woman who has been diagnosed with an intrauterine fetal demise (IUFD):

   a. Delivery should be induced as soon as possible to reduce the risk for intrauterine infection

   b. Parents should be offered the option of labor induction or waiting for spontaneous labor

    c. Waiting for spontaneous labor allows the parents to have a more healthy grieving process

    d. There is a high risk for maternal coagulopathy within the first week after fetal demise

82. Risks associated with post-term pregnancy include:

    a. Macrosomia, meconium aspiration, polyhydramnios

    b. Growth retardation, pre-eclampsia, oligohydramnios

    c. Macrosomia, increased risk for C-section delivery, placental insufficiency

    d. Pre-eclampsia, meconium aspiration, oligohydramnios

83. A 16-year-old client who is 37-weeks-pregnant is admitted to the hospital with severe pre-eclampsia. Magnesium sulfate ($MgSO_4$) is ordered. The primary reason for administering $MgSO_4$ to this client is to:

    a. Increase urinary output

    b. Lower blood pressure

    c. Prevent seizure activity

    d. Promote uterine relaxation

84. During assessment of the client on $MgSO_4$, a sign of developing toxicity would be:

    a. Headache with blurred vision

    b. Increased deep tendon reflexes

    c. Severe right upper quadrant pain

    d. Urinary output less than 30 mL/hr

85. The antidote for $MgSO_4$ toxicity is:

    a. Betamethasone

    b. Calcium gluconate

    c. Nifedipine

    d. Propranolol

86. A 40-year-old woman presents for her initial prenatal visit 12 weeks from her LNMP. She is complaining of severe nausea with vomiting and some vaginal spotting. On examination her fundus is at the umbilicus and there are no fetal heart tones. In addition, her blood pressure is 154/106 mm Hg. The most likely diagnosis for this woman is:

    a. Hydatidiform mole

    b. Missed abortion

c. Multiple gestation

d. Polyhydramnios

87. A 37-year-old, G3 P2 woman presents at 34.5 weeks gestation. Her pregnancy has been complicated by chronic hypertension with superimposed pre-eclampsia. She received late prenatal care because she was incarcerated for drug charges and has a long history of cocaine and tobacco use. The medical plan is to deliver her as soon as fetal lung maturity has been demonstrated. Given her history, you would expect:

a. Accelerated lung maturity in this fetus

b. Delayed lung maturity in this fetus

c. An inaccurate lecithin/sphingomyelin (L/S) ratio in this patient

d. An inaccurate phosphatidylglycerol (PG) ratio in this patient

88. A 36-year-old primipara presents with her LNMP 14 weeks ago. She complains of fatigue, backache, and nausea and vomiting all day. She is 5' 6'' and weighs 140 pounds. Her vital signs and physical examination are within normal limits. Fundal height is two fingerbreadths below the umbilicus. Fetal heart tones are present. Routine prenatal laboratory tests are ordered. Other prenatal care for this client should include:

a. Scheduling her to return in one to two weeks for an MSAFP

b. Obtaining an MSAFP at this visit and having her return in four weeks

c. Scheduling an ultrasound and ordering a quantitative hCG

d. Scheduling her for an ultrasound as soon as possible

89. Potential complications for twin gestation include:

a. Preterm labor, hyperemesis, and gestational diabetes

b. Cord accidents, congenital anomalies, and thrombophlebitis

c. Congenital anomalies, placenta previa, and postpartum hemorrhage

d. Anemia, thrombophlebitis, cord accidents, and gallstones

90. Healthy twins, one girl and one boy, are delivered at 36 weeks gestation. You send the placenta to pathology. What report would you expect to get back?

a. Monochorionic-monoamniotic

b. Monochorionic-diamniotic

c. Dichorionic-diamniotic

d. Dichorionic-monoamniotic

Questions 91, 92, and 93 refer to the following scenario.

An 18-year-old pregnant client who has received no prenatal care presents to the labor and delivery unit on August 6th contracting every five minutes for 50 seconds. The contractions are moderate to strong to palpation. She states that her last period was ''for sure'' on New Year's Day. Fundal height is 31 cm with the fetus in the vertex position. A nonstress test is reactive.

91. The next assessment that should be done is a:

    a. Biophysical profile
    b. Sterile digital examination
    c. Sterile speculum examination
    d. Transvaginal ultrasound

92. During assessment of this client several genital specimens were obtained. The test that requires a specimen from the outer one third of the vagina is the:

    a. Fern patttern test
    b. Fibronectin assay
    c. Nitrazine pH test
    d. Group B streptococcus culture

93. A decision has been made to initiate tocolytic therapy. The physician has also ordered the administration of betamethasone IM. This is done because administration of corticosteroids:

    a. Decreases possible respiratory side effects of tocolytic drugs
    b. Decreases the incidence of premature rupture of membranes
    c. Enhances the ability of tocolytics to prolong pregnancy
    d. Reduces the incidence of newborn respiratory distress syndrome

94. The tocolytic agent terbutaline is administered to stop preterm labor. Maternal complications with this medication include:

    a. Pulmonary edema
    b. Hypertension
    c. Respiratory depression
    d. Severe bronchospasms

95. On examining a woman who had a normal spontaneous vaginal delivery eight hours ago you would expect to find the fundus:

a. At the umbilicus, the vagina gaping, and bright red bleeding on the perineal pad
b. 3/4 of the way between the symphysis and umbilicus, the vagina edematous, and bright red bleeding on the perineal pad
c. 1 to 2 fingerbreadths above the umbilicus, the vagina gaping, and serous vaginal bleeding on the pad
d. 1 to 2 fingerbreadths below the umbilicus, the vagina edematous, and serous vaginal bleeding on the pad

96. 16 hours after a normal spontaneous vaginal delivery a woman has a WBC count of 20,000 mm^3. She also has a temperature of 100.2° F. These findings are indicative of:

a. Milk production
b. Normal postpartum
c. Retained placental fragments
d. Urinary tract infection

97. For the woman who chooses not to breast feed, advice on enhancing suppression of lactation and decreasing discomfort would include:

a. Apply warm compresses to the breasts every four hours
b. Consider the use of prolactin inhibiting medication
c. Avoid wearing a brassiere as this will stimulate the nipples
d. Avoid letting shower water flow over the breasts

98. In discussing postpartum contraception with a woman prior to her delivery, the information you give her is based on your knowledge that she may regain her fertility prior to:

a. Her six weeks checkup so she should use some form of contraception when she resumes intercourse
b. Her first menses but she should not need contraception before her six weeks checkup
c. Her six weeks checkup only if she resumes menstruation before that time
d. Her six weeks checkup but most women choose not to resume intercourse before then

99. Information for the breast feeding woman who is considering the lactational amenorrhea method (LAM) for contraception should include telling her that:

a. As long as she breast feeds on demand and remains amenorrheic this method is considered 98% effective

b. This method is 98% effective for the first six months if she nurses on demand, rarely gives supplements, and remains amenorrheic
c. As long as she nurses on demand and provides no supplements this method is considered 98% effective
d. LAM is not a highly effective method of contraception so she should consider other contraception after 6 to 8 weeks postpartum

100. When counseling the breast feeding mother concerning infant nutrition, she should be told that:

a. Iron fortified cereal or liquid iron should be started at about three months of age
b. The concentration of iron in breast milk is generally higher than that in formula
c. The infant should need no form of iron supplementation for the first 4 to 6 months
d. If a fluoride supplement is used, it should be given along with an iron supplement

101. An examination of a 6-weeks-postpartum client reveals a uterus that is approximately eight week size, soft, and nontender. Her temperature is 98.4° F. She has had irregular, heavy bleeding for the past two weeks. She states that she has not had sexual intercourse since her delivery. These findings are indicative of:

a. A normal postpartum course
b. A resolving uterine hematoma
c. Postpartum endometritis
d. Subinvolution of the uterus

102. A 23-year-old client who is four hours post normal spontaneous vaginal delivery of her first child has a small, second degree laceration which was repaired without difficulty. She has no complicating factors. To help with perineal discomfort you instruct her to:

a. Apply ice packs to her perineum for the first 24 hours then sitz baths
b Apply hot packs to her perineum for the first 24 hours then ice as needed
c. Apply ice packs intermittently with warm sitz baths for the first 24 hours
d. Apply an analgesic cream to her perineal area as needed

103. A 32-year-old G3 P3 who delivered an 8 lb 10 oz infant one week ago calls today complaining of backache and bright red vaginal bleeding. She states she is soaking a pad an hour. Given her history you:

    a. Recognize that this is most likely due to excess physical activity
    b. Suspect that she is having her first postpartum menstrual period
    c. Consider that she may have retained placental fragments
    d. Suspect that she had extensive perineal lacerations during delivery

104. A 21-year-old woman delivered her first baby five weeks ago. She had a normal spontaneous delivery after 14 hours of labor and 30 hours of ruptured membranes. Her postpartum course has been unremarkable. She has been breast feeding her infant on demand since birth and has had some problems with cracked nipples, but otherwise is satisfied with how well it is going. She calls the office today with the complaint of a headache, flu like symptoms, a tenderness on her right breast, and a temperature of 103° F. Management should include:

    a. Advising extra fluids and bedrest until her temperature returns to normal
    b. Initiating antibiotics and advising her to discontinue breastfeeding for 48 hours
    c. Advising her she will need to be admitted to the hospital for IV antibiotics
    d. Initiating antibiotics and advising her to take extra fluids and to nurse frequently

105. During childbirth preparation class a mother asks about the benefits and risks of epidural anesthesia. An appropriate response would include telling her that:

    a. Small amounts of anesthetic are absorbed into the bloodstream so there is a risk for fetal hypotension
    b. Maternal hypotension is a possible complication and this may lead to fetal bradycardia
    c. Studies have shown that the use of epidural anesthesia often leads to a faster progression of labor
    d. Prior to epidural anesthesia a catheter is inserted in the bladder to prevent urinary retention

106. Which of the following statements concerning postpartum depression is true?

    a. It may occur any time during the first postpartum year
    b. The woman who has a premature baby is at increased risk
    c. Postpartum depression usually improves without any treatment
    d. If untreated, postpartum depression often leads to psychosis

107. Which of the following statements is most true regarding attachment and bonding between parents and babies?

a. The presence of the family at the time of birth has been shown to be a strong factor in establishing a strong bond between infant and mother
b. There are three sequential time periods during which attachment and bonding between parents and baby develop and take place
c. The presence of a long labor decreases the strength of the attachment
d. Use of anesthesia/analgesia in labor has been shown to have a positive effect on maternal infant bonding

108. In childbirth class you are discussing options for pain relief in labor. A couple asks about a pudendal block. You tell them this is a technique of injecting:

a. Local anesthetic into the subcutaneous tissue of the perineum to numb the area prior to episiotomy
b. An anesthetic into the caudal space in the spine to cause a numbing of the perineal area
c. An anesthetic transvaginally just prior to birth to numb the perineum and lower vagina
d. Regional anesthetic into the epidural space to provide relief from the pain of contractions

Answers and Rationale

1. **(a)** Elevated progesterone levels cause smooth muscle relaxation resulting in decreased peristalsis. This contributes to the common complaint of constipation during pregnancy (Ladewig, et al., p. 155).

2. **(c)** A prepregnant weight of 130 lbs. for a woman who is 5' 6'' would be considered within normal limits. Recommended weight gain for the woman of normal weight is 25 to 35 lbs. A woman who is underweight (< 90% of ideal body weight) should gain 28 to 40 pounds, and a woman who is obese (> 120% of ideal body weight) should gain 15 to 25 lbs. (Varney, p. 321).

3. **(b)** The expected level of the fundus at 12 weeks is the symphysis pubis, at 16 weeks $\frac{1}{2}$ way between the symphysis pubis and umbilicus, and at 20 weeks the umbilicus (Varney, p. 732).

4. **(b)** Heartburn is a common discomfort in the late second and third trimesters. Relaxation of the cardiac sphincter and decreased gastrointestinal motility contribute to heartburn. In addition, there is less room for the stomach to expand due to the increasing size of the uterus. Small, frequent meals may help to prevent heartburn by preventing overload of the stomach. Beverages should be avoided during meals as they tend to inhibit gastric juices. Lying down immediately after eating increases the likelihood for gastric reflux. Low sodium antacids may be used (Ladewig, et al., p. 204; Varney, p. 268).

5. **(a)** Presumptive signs of pregnancy are physiological changes the woman experiences that suggest to her that she may be pregnant. Probable signs of pregnancy are maternal physiological and anatomical changes other than presumptive signs that indicate to her she is pregnant. Positive signs are those directly attributable to the fetus as detected and documented by a trained examiner such at the palpation of fetal movement and viewing the fetus on ultrasound (Varney, p. 229).

6. **(c)** At the end of the first trimester, both components of the first heart sound become louder and there is an exaggerated splitting due to the increased circulating blood volume (Gabbe, et al., p. 162).

7. **(d)** G6 T3 P1 A1 L2. Gravida is any pregnancy, regardless of duration, including the present pregnancy. Term is delivery at 38 to 42 weeks gestation. Preterm is delivery after 20 weeks but before completion of 37 weeks gestation. Spontaneous abortion refers to expulsion of the fetus prior to viability. Stillbirth refers to an infant born dead after 20 weeks gestation. A stillbirth at 34 weeks gestation would be considered a premature birth (Ladewig, et al., p. 171).

8. **(d)** hCG is produced by the trophoblast and is first detectable in the urine about 26 days after conception or in the blood about seven days after conception (Varney, p. 231).

9. **(a)** TSH levels remain within the normal, nonpregnant range during pregnancy. There is an estrogen induced increase in TBG. The increase in TBG results in an increase in total T_4 and T_3 levels. Concentrations of active thyroid hormones (free T_4 and T_3) do not change during pregnancy (Gabbe, et al., p. 104).

10. **(d)** Using Nagele's rule, one takes the first day of the last menstrual period, adds seven days and then subtracts three months to get an EDD. 11/20 plus seven days = 11/27, minus three months = 8/27 (Varney, p. 255).

11. **(b)** The pregnant woman with a positive PPD test should have a chest radiograph. An abdominal shield should be used to protect the fetus from radiation. Treatment regimens are determined by the results of the chest radiograph and by timing of seroconversion if known (Hauth & Merenstein, pp. 238-239).

12. **(c)** ACOG guidelines recommend that starting women on prophylactic zidovudine (ZVD) therapy between 14 and 34 weeks gestation can significantly decrease the rate of mother to infant transmission. This prophylaxis is continued through labor and delivery and the infant is administered ZVD orally every six hours for the first six weeks of life. Currently there is no definitive data on the role of C-section in reducing perinatal transmission, but recommendations are that membranes not be artificially ruptured, scalp electrodes not be placed, and scalp pH not be measured unless absolutely necessary (Hauth & Merenstein, pp. 219-220; Gabbe, et al., p. 1224).

13. **(d)** Chloasma, or the "mask of pregnancy" is an irregular brownish discoloration of the forehead, cheeks, and nose. It is believed to be the result of the melanocyte stimulating effect of estrogen and progesterone. This discoloration usually fades and disappears after pregnancy has ended (Varney, p. 230).

14. **(a)** hPL stimulates growth of the breasts and has lactogenic properties in addition to having a number of metabolic effects (Varney, p. 230).

15. **(c)** Softening of the uterine isthmus (Hegar's sign) is evident at about six weeks gestation. Braxton-Hicks contractions may start as early as six weeks gestation, but are not palpable with bimanual examination until the second trimester. As the uterus becomes an abdominal organ it rotates slightly to the right (dextrorotation). The uterus is palpable at the symphysis pubis at 12 weeks gestation (Varney, pp. 232-233).

16. **(d)** Softening of the ligaments of the pubic symphysis and sacroiliac joints occur due to the effects of the hormone relaxin. This hormone also inhibits uterine activity and aids in the softening of the cervix (Gabbe, et al., p. 100; Ladewig, et al., p. 157).

17. **(b)** Hemodynamic changes that occur during pregnancy include increased cardiac output, decreased systemic vascular resistance, and increased heart rate (Gabbe, et al., p. 99).

18. **(c)** A clean catch urine sample showing the presence of 50,000 pathogenic bacteria of the same species per mL most often indicates an infection. Because untreated asymptomatic bacteriuria is associated with pyelonephritis, preterm labor, and low birth weight, it should be treated with the appropriate antibiotic. A repeat urine culture two weeks after treatment should be considered to assure that antibiotic therapy was effective (Varney, pp. 343-344).

19. **(c)** Leg cramps are a common discomfort in the third trimester of pregnancy. The exact cause is unknown. Changes in calcium and phosphorus metabolism and pressure from the enlarging uterus on pelvic nerves and blood vessels are possible causes. Dorsiflexing the foot is helpful as this stretches

the calf muscle. Walking promotes circulation and stretches the calf muscles as long as high heeled shoes are avoided. The woman can either decrease milk intake and add a calcium carbonate supplement, or maintain her current milk intake and take aluminum hydroxide gel with meals to absorb phosphorus. Either of these dietary changes is intended to correct or prevent calcium phosphorus imbalance (Ladewig, et al., p. 206).

20. **(c)** Current recommendations are that women should take 0.4 mg of folic acid daily both before conception and during the first trimester to help prevent neural tube defects. Women with a history of a previous pregnancy with a neural tube defect should begin taking 4 mg of folic acid daily for the month prior to conception and during the first trimester (Hauth & Merenstein, p. 280).

21. **(c)** The blastocyst develops into the embryo, amnion, and yolk sac membrane (Varney, p. 238).

22. **(b)** The most highly sensitive time for a teratogenic effect on the heart is between weeks 3 to 7. The entire embryonic period is a critical time for teratogenesis that may be lethal or cause major congenital malformations (Varney, pp. 241-242).

23. **(b)** The corpus luteum is responsible for secreting progesterone to prevent endometrial shedding (menses). It remains functional until about the 12th week when the placenta takes over the function of secreting progesterone (Varney, pp. 229-230).

24. **(a)** The WBC count rises throughout pregnancy. The average WBC count is 9,500 mm^3 in the first trimester, 10,500 mm^3 in the second and third trimesters, and 20,000 to 30,000 mm^3 during labor and delivery. It returns to normal by the end of the first week postpartum. Hematocrit, platelet count, and serum ferritin may all be lower in pregnancy (Gabbe, et al., p. 102).

25. **(c)** There is no evidence of fetal risk from toxoid vaccines such as the tetanus vaccine or from tetanus immune globulin. Recommendations are to administer a booster if more than five years have elapsed since the last dose with this type of wound (Gabbe, et al., p. 177; DHHS, p. 368).

26. **(c)** An IgG varicella serology can be done to confirm immune status. If it is positive the woman can be assured that her fetus is not at risk (Gabbe, et al., p. 1238).

27. **(a)** Amniocentesis may be used to detect chromosomal disorders, Rh sensitization, fetal lung maturity, and amnionitis. It is not useful in detecting birth defects caused by teratogens (Hauth & Merenstein, pp. 77-78).

28. **(c)** The results of a nonstress test are considered reassuring when there is a minimum of two or more accelerations in the fetal heart rate of 15 or more beats for 15 or more seconds in a 20 minute period (Hauth & Merenstein, p. 86).

29. **(d)** Vena cava syndrome or supine hypotension occurs when the pregnant woman lies in a supine position, because of the weight of the uterus and fetus on the inferior vena cava. The woman may feel dizzy, light headed and may even have syncope. Symptoms can be alleviated by having the woman turn on her side (Varney, p. 273; Gabbe, et al., p. 98).

30. **(d)** A biophysical profile (BPP) of 6 out of 10 with a normal amniotic fluid volume is considered to be equivocal. If the fetus is mature, delivery is indicated. If the fetus is not mature the BPP should be repeated within 24 hours (Varney, p. 304).

31. **(c)** Although there are several different counting methods, most commonly the woman has one count session at the same time each day. It may be useful to schedule her count session about one hour after a meal while resting on her left side to promote uteroplacental circulation. She should contact her health care provider if she feels less than 10 movements in one hour or if it takes longer to count 10 movements than is usual for her (Youngkin & Davis, p. 607).

32. **(a)** Bishop scoring is done to evaluate cervical readiness for induction. The five factors evaluated include dilatation, effacement, station, cervix consistency, and cervix position (Varney, p. 473).

33. **(d)** The monitor strip shows late decelerations. This type of deceleration is most commonly seen with uteroplacental insufficiency. Early decelerations

may be seen with head compression and are usually benign. Variable decelerations are seen with cord compression. A temporary sinusoidal pattern may be seen in association with analgesic medication (Ladewig, et al., pp. 384-385).

34. **(d)** Positioning a woman on her left side will increase the blood flow to the uterus. Administering oxygen at 6 to 8 liters/minute will increase the amount available to the fetus between contractions. Hydration should be maintained with an IV and if oxytocin is being administered it should be discontinued (Ladewig, et al., p. 388).

35. **(d)** A negative contraction stress test (CST) indicates there were no late decelerations with adequate uterine contractions (3 in 10 minutes). A negative CST has consistently been associated with good fetal outcome. It is considered to be predictive for seven days so weekly retesting is appropriate when using the CST to screen for uteroplacental insufficiency (Gabbe, et al., p. 337; Varney, p. 300).

36. **(c)** The vaginal examination findings of 50%, 3 cm, -1 describe a cervix that is 50% effaced, 3 cm dilated, and fetal presenting part that is 1 cm (-1 station) above the ischial spines. The fetal presenting part is considered floating when it is at −5 station (Varney, p. 385).

37. **(b)** Implantation occurs between days 7 and 9 after fertilization. An abortion is classified as inevitable when there is cervical dilatation or rupture of membranes. With an incomplete abortion the internal os will be dilated slightly and bleeding is often profuse. This client's symptoms and physical examination findings may be indicative of either a threatened abortion or an ectopic pregnancy (Varney, pp. 328-329, 332).

38. **(c)** hCG levels double about every 48 hours in a normal intrauterine pregnancy (Ladewig, et al., p. 285).

39. **(b)** CDC treatment guidelines state that podophyllin, podofilox and imiquimod should not be used during pregnancy. Treatment during pregnancy with trichloroacetic acid or cryotherapy may be considered as genital warts often proliferate and become friable during pregnancy (CDC, p. 93).

40. **(d)** Although a false positive hCG may occur, it may be indicative of an hCG secreting tumor of the pancreas, ovary or breast (Pagana & Pagana, p. 351).

41. **(a)** For an infant to have sickle cell disease, both parents must have the trait and the child must inherit the trait from both parents. With an autosomal recessive trait, this is a one in four chance (Ladewig, et al., p. 82).

42. **(a)** The most accurate measurement is in the first trimester where the CRL +/- value is only five days in 95% of cases. Biparietal diameter at 20 weeks gestation has a +/- value of 12 days. Femur length at 30 weeks gestation has a +/- value of 11 days. Abdominal circumference is used in combination with other parameters for evaluation of fetal growth in the third trimester (Gabbe, et al., pp. 284-286).

43. **(a)** Information concerning chromosomal status and DNA patterns can be obtained through chorionic villi sampling (CVS). Information that requires amniotic fluid, such as an alpha-fetoprotein (AFP) to detect neural tube abnormalities cannot be obtained. Studies concerning limb reduction defects related to CVS indicate that the greatest risk is associated with the procedure performed at less than 10 weeks gestation. Pregnancy loss rates with CVS have been shown to be no different from loss rates after amniocentesis (Gabbe, et al., pp. 228-231).

44. **(c)** Chronic hypertension is considered to be one of the many risk factors for intrauterine growth retardation (IUGR). Other risk factors include low maternal prepregnancy weight (< 90% IBW), poor maternal weight gain, diabetes mellitus, substance abuse, maternal anemia (Hgb < 10 g/dL), multiple gestation, and abnormalities of the placenta (Varney, pp. 866-867).

45. **(c)** When excessive fetomaternal bleeding is a concern with an Rh negative client, a Kliehauer-Betke test can be used to determine the volume of fetal red blood cells in the maternal circulation. The appropriate dose of Rh immune globulin to be given can be calculated according to the results of this test (Gabbe, et al., pp. 905-906).

46. **(c)** Methotrexate is a folic acid antagonist that interferes with DNA synthesis and cell multiplication (Gabbe, et al., p. 734).

47. **(b)** Because methotrexate is a folic acid antagonist, the client should avoid any supplements containing folic acid during treatment (Gabbe, et al., p. 734).

48. **(d)** Most women can continue to exercise safely during pregnancy with some precautions. Running is an acceptable form of exercise during pregnancy if the woman is already in a regular running program and not having any problems with the pregnancy. Precautions include limiting exercise sessions to no more than 60 minutes to reduce any risk of fetal hyperthermia, stopping exercise if she feels fatigued, keeping heart rate at about 60% to 75% of maximal heart rate, not exercising in hot weather, and attending to hydration. She should also exercise 3 or 4 times a week as layoffs followed by quick returns increase the risk for injury. Caloric intake needed is directly influenced by a woman's activity level. She must monitor her weight gain to assure that she is getting adequate calories (Carlson & Parrish, pp. 172, 174-175).

49. **(d)** This client's risk factors for placental abruption include smoking, hypertension, poor weight gain, and maternal age over 35. Signs and symptoms of placental abruption may include bleeding (although it may be concealed), back pain, colicky abdominal pain, and increased uterine tone between contractions. Depending on the degree of separation there may be abnormalities in fetal heart rate pattern, a decrease or absence of fetal activity, and signs of maternal shock (Varney, pp. 366-367).

50. **(d)** Ultrasound provides for evaluation of the fetus, placenta and uterus. Continuous fetal monitoring for at least four hours should occur to observe for signs of decreased long term variability indicating fetal stress, and for signs of uterine tetany and/or late decelerations. Since placental abruption frequently stimulates the clotting cascade resulting in DIC, coagulation studies including fibrinogen, platelet count, PT, and PTT should be measured (Gabbe, et al., pp. 506-507).

51. **(a)** Risk factors for placental abruption include hypertension, pre-eclampsia, folic acid deficiency, abdominal trauma, short umbilical cord, malnutrition, sudden decrease in uterine volume, maternal age over 35, difficult or rough version, smoking, and cocaine or crack usage (Varney, p. 366).

52. **(c)** HELLP stands for Hemolysis, Elevated Liver enzymes, and Low Platelets. These are the physiologic abnormalities that may be seen with progressive pre-eclampsia (Varney, p. 363).

53. **(b)** Pre-eclampsia is characterized by the development of an elevated BP ($\geq$ 140/90 mm Hg or systolic rise $\geq$ 30 mm Hg or diastolic rise $\geq$ 15 mm Hg above baseline), with proteinuria and/or generalized edema after 20 weeks gestation (Varney, p. 359).

54. **(d)** Risk factors for asymptomatic bacteriuria in pregnancy include a history of urinary tract infections, diabetes, and sickle cell trait/disease. Untreated asymptomatic bacteriuria is associated with pyelonephritis, preterm delivery and low birth weight (Varney, p. 345)

55. **(a)** The placental hormones, (estrogen, progesterone, and especially hPL) interfere with the action of maternal insulin. hPL levels rise 10 fold in the second half of pregnancy (Gabbe, et al., p. 105).

56. **(c)** ACOG recommendations are that either universal or selective screening for gestational diabetes be performed at 24 to 28 weeks of gestation. For selective screening the following risk factors may be used: Family history of diabetes, previous birth of macrosomic, malformed or stillbirth baby, hypertension, glycosuria, maternal age of > 30 years, or previous gestational diabetes (Hauth & Merenstein, p. 77).

57. **(c)** The diagnosis of gestational diabetes is made when any two of the following glucose values on plasma samples are met or exceeded: Fasting—105 mg, 1 hour—190 mg, 2 hour—165 mg, 3 hour—145 mg (Gabbe, et al., p. 1048).

58. **(a)** The glycosylated hemoglobin (Hgb A_{1c}) provides an accurate long term index of the client's average blood glucose over the previous 8 to 12 weeks. This would be useful in helping the client to obtain strict control of her glucose levels prior to pregnancy. Strict diabetes control prior to pregnancy and early in pregnancy may reduce the risk for congenital anomalies that are more common with maternal diabetes. Oral hypoglycemics are contraindicated during pregnancy. The need for insulin frequently decreases in the

first trimester and then begins to rise in the second trimester. Fetal macrosomia results when there are high levels of maternal glucose. Strict glucose control during pregnancy may reduce this risk (Ladewig, et al., pp. 260-262).

59. **(d)** Vitamin B_{12} occurs naturally only in foods of animal origin. A vitamin B_{12} supplement should be provided for women who eat no meat products. Folic acid is found in green, leafy vegetables. Iron may be obtained by eating whole grains, enriched breads and cereals, dark green leafy vegetables, and dried fruits. Protein is found in dairy products, grains, and legumes (Ludwig, et al., pp. 243-245).

60. **(b)** Aspirin decreases platelet aggregation which can increase the risk of bleeding before and during delivery. There is also some risk of premature closure of the fetal ductus arteriosis with the prostoglandin synthetase inhibitors such as aspirin, ibuprofen, and naproxen. Acetaminophen use does not have these potential adverse effects and is preferred when a mild analgesic or antipyretic is indicated. A nasal decongestant is preferred to an oral decongestant as topical administration results in a lower dose to the fetus (Gabbe, et al., pp. 260-263).

61. **(c)** The indirect Coombs test (antibody screen) determines if the mother has any antibodies to Rh positive blood. The test is routinely done for Rh negative women at their initial visit and at 27 to 28 weeks. If the test is positive it indicates that the mother has already been sensitized. RhoGAM is used to prevent sensitization but does not reverse pre-existing sensitization. If the baby is Rh negative, RhoGAM is not needed. Therefore it is the mother with a negative indirect Coombs and an Rh positive baby who will benefit from receiving RhoGAM after delivery (Ladewig, et al., p. 308).

62. **(a)** Kell refers to the K or K1 antigen of the Kell blood group system. About 0.2% of pregnant women are positive for anti-Kell with nearly all cases of isoimmunization occurring as a result of a Kell-incompatible transfusion. Kell isoimmunization can result in erythroblastosis fetalis. RhoGAM is not effective in preventing Kell isoimmunization (Gabbe, et al., p. 922).

63. **(c)** ABO incompatibility is a common cause of hemolytic disease in the newborn. However, it rarely results in severe hemolytic disease with less than 1% requiring exchange transfusions. It usually manifests itself as mild to

moderate hyperbilirubinemia during the first 24 to 48 hours of life. ABO incompatibility occurs when the mother's blood type is O and the infant's blood type is A or B (Gabbe, et al., p. 923).

64. **(b)** Spectrophotometric analysis of amniotic fluid bilirubin levels correlate with the severity of fetal hemolysis in Rh isoimmunization. The Liley graph (optical density graph) is used to plot the serial measurement of bilirubin in the amniotic fluid as determined by spectrophotometry. The results on the graph are used to place the fetus in zones representing unaffected to severely affected. The graph is used to help clinicians in making decisions about the timing of delivery (Gabbe, et al., p. 908).

65. **(b)** MSAFP is designed as a screening test to be administered between 15 and 22 weeks gestation. Results are most accurate when performed between 16 and 18 weeks. The most common reason for a false positive is incorrect dates. Undiagnosed multiple gestation may also cause a false positive. If the results come back abnormal, ultrasound should be scheduled. The ultrasound will help in determining an accurate gestational date or presence of multiple gestations (ACOG, 1996b, pp. 3-5).

66. **(b)** FAS (fetal alcohol syndrome) is now believed to be the number one preventable birth defect. Down syndrome and some neural tube defects may be genetic based, and IUGR is not a birth defect (Ladewig, et al., p. 274).

67. **(c)** Serial cervical and vaginal cultures have not been shown to be predictive for newborn infection. The benefits of prophylactic administration of acyclovir have not been established. Routine Cesarean delivery is not recommended. Cesarean delivery is recommended if a lesion is present that cannot be covered or is in an area that the baby might come in contact with during delivery (Hauth & Merenstein, p. 214).

68. **(b)** Rubella vaccine is not recommended during pregnancy because it is an attenuated live virus. To avoid risk, women should be advised to avoid pregnancy for three months after receiving the vaccine. However, no evidence of teratogenicity from the vaccine has been demonstrated (Varney, p. 340).

69. **(c)** TORCH is an acronym for a variety of infections that may cause harm to the fetus during pregnancy. It stands for Toxoplasmosis, Other infections,

Rubella, Cytomegalovirus inclusion disease and Herpes (Hauth & Merenstein, p. 207).

70. **(c)** About 50% of women are immune to fifth disease (human parvovirus) but even with close exposure the highest risk of contracting the disease is 50%. There is a low risk of ill effects on the fetus. Most infections that have resulted in fetal death occurred in the first half of pregnancy. Third trimester infections have been associated with anemia in the newborn (Hauth & Merenstein, p. 222).

71. **(b)** Polyhydramnios is associated with diabetes, GI tract anomalies, neural tube defects, Rh isoimmunization, and multiple gestations. Potential complications with polyhydramnios include preterm labor, placental abruption, prolapsed cord with rupture of membranes, and postpartum hemorrhage because of uterine overdistention (Ladewig, et al., p. 473).

72. **(c)** Oligohydramnios is associated with major fetal renal malformations. It may also be found with post-term pregnancy and with IUGR that is secondary to placental insufficiency (Ladewig, et. al., p. 474).

73. **(a)** Nitrazine paper may turn blue in the presence of blood, some cervical secretions, and some vaginal infections in addition to amniotic fluid. Cervical secretions will frequently dry in a fern pattern so fluid must be obtained from the posterior fornix for the most accurate reading. Fluid seen escaping from the cervical os is diagnostic for ruptured membranes (Varney, p. 390).

74. **(a)** Contraction frequency is timed from the beginning of one contraction to the beginning of the next contraction (Ladewig, et al., p. 344).

75. **(c)** Second degree lacerations include the vaginal mucosa, posterior fourchette, perineal skin, and perineal muscles (Varney, p. 864).

76. **(c)** The first stage of labor is defined as beginning with true labor contractions, which cause progressive cervical dilatation and ending with the cervix being completely dilated (Varney, p. 395).

77. **(a)** ACOG recommendations are that the FHR should be evaluated at least every 30 minutes just after a contraction in the active phase of the first stage of labor, and at least every 15 minutes during the second stage of labor in someone with no risk factors (Hauth & Merenstein, p. 101).

78. **(d)** The basic positional movements in the normal mechanism of labor are engagement, descent, flexion, internal rotation, restitution, and external rotation (Varney, p. 436).

79. **(b)** VBAC contraindications include circumstances that would place the woman at high risk for uterine rupture. A trial of labor should not be attempted if a) there was a prior classical or T-shaped uterine incision, b) there is a contracted pelvis, c) there is a medical or obstetric complication precluding vaginal delivery or d) if there is not the capability to perform an immediate emergency C-section if needed. Given this client's history of "a little extra cut" on the uterine incision, she most likely had a classical or T-shaped incision (ACOG, 1998, p. 3).

80. **(b)** Signs and symptoms of intrauterine fetal demise (IUFD) include cessation of fetal movement and heart tones, cessation of uterine growth, and Spalding's sign (excessive overlapping of the skull bones) on ultrasound or radiograph. The sudden increase in fetal activity followed by cessation of movement is an ominous sign (Varney, p. 358).

81. **(b)** The woman/couple should be encouraged to make as many choices as possible about medical care including the timing of delivery. Most women choose to be delivered as soon as possible, however it is acceptable to wait until spontaneous labor begins (usually within 2 to 3 weeks of fetal death) as long as coagulation studies are done each week to screen for DIC. Coagulopathy does not usually occur unless a dead fetus has been retained longer than four weeks (Varney, p. 359; Hauth & Merenstein, pp. 200-201).

82. **(c)** Risks associated with post-term pregnancy include macrosomia, increased chance of operative delivery, meconium aspiration, placental insufficiency, and oligohydramnios (Gabbe, et al., pp. 888-890).

83. **(c)** Magnesium sulfate ($MgSO_4$) acts as a CNS depressant. Its primary use with severe pre-eclampsia is seizure prevention. Because it secondarily relaxes smooth muscle, it may also reduce blood pressure and decrease the frequency and intensity of contractions (Ladewig, et al., p. 293).

84. **(d)** Signs of developing $MgSO_4$ toxicity include depression or absence of reflexes, oliguria, confusion, and respiratory depression (Ladewig, et al., p. 293).

85. **(b)** The antidote for $MgSO_4$ toxicity is calcium gluconate (Ladewig, et al., p. 293).

86. **(a)** Hydatidiform moles occur most frequently in older women, especially those older than 40 years. Symptoms usually occur before the 18th week of amenorrhea and include vaginal bleeding, hyperemesis gravidarum, and pregnancy induced hypertension. In 50% of cases the uterus is large for gestational dates (Niswander & Evans, p. 460).

87. **(a)** Accelerated lung maturity is associated with hypertensive disorders, hemoglobinopathies, narcotic addiction, IUGR, PROM, multiple gestation, and smoking (ACOG, 1996a, p. 5).

88. **(d)** The most common presentation for a twin gestation is a large for dates uterus and prolonged nausea and vomiting. A woman may also complain of early or excessive fetal movement, and two fetal heart tones may be auscultated. Another reason for excessive nausea and vomiting and increased fundal height may also be a hydatidiform mole. The distinction would be uterine bleeding by the 12th week and no fetal heart tones. The initial step in this situation would be to obtain an ultrasound. Accurate gestational dating and determination of multiple gestation are important prior to an MSAFP (Varney, p. 356)

89. **(c)** Potential complication for the fetus in a multiple gestation pregnancy include SGA, IUGR, cord accidents, malpresentation, congenital anomalies, and twin to twin transfusion. For the mother, potential complications include PIH, placenta previa, preterm labor and postpartum hemorrhage (Gabbe, et al., p. 823; Varney, p. 356).

90. **(c)** Delivery of a girl and boy tells you they are dizygotic or fraternal twins. Dizygotic twins always have dichorionic-diamniotic placentas although they may be fused (Ladewig, et al., p. 44).

91. **(c)** Sterile speculum examination should be performed to evaluate membrane status and to obtain cultures for group B streptococcus, chlamydia and gonorrhea. Digital examination should only be performed after rupture of membranes has been ruled out. Transabdominal ultrasound may be useful in confirming gestational age. A biophysical profile might be indicated if the nonstress test was nonreactive (Gabbe, et al., p. 764).

92. **(d)** The specimen for the group B streptococcus culture should be obtained from the outer one third of the vagina and the perineum. The specimen for the fern pattern test should be obtained from fluid in the posterior vaginal fornix or from fluid coming out of the cervical os. The specimen for pH testing can be obtained from the blade of the speculum to obtain fluid from the posterior fornix. A specimen taken from the cervical os may produce a false positive color change because cervical mucus may be alkaline. The specimen for the fibronectin assay should be obtained from the external cervical os and the posterior fornix (Varney, pp. 467-468; Gabbe, et al., p. 764).

93. **(d)** Administration of corticosteroids to women between 24 and 34 weeks gestation has been demonstrated to induce fetal lung maturity and to decrease the chance of intraventricular hemorrhage and respiratory distress syndrome (ACOG, 1996a, p. 230).

94. **(a)** Terbutaline is a beta adrenergic agonist. It stimulates the beta receptors resulting in smooth muscle relaxation. Pulmonary edema is the most serious complication with the use of terbutaline. Other side effects include tachycardia, hypotension, hyperglycemia, hypokalemia, and jitteriness (Gabbe, et al., p. 769).

95. **(a)** Lochia rubra is bright red and is seen for the first 2 to 3 days postpartum. Immediately after delivery the vagina appears stretched and bruised with some edema. The fundus should be at the umbilicus within a few hours of delivery. If it is above the umbilicus consider that it may be due to filling of the uterus with blood clots or displacement by a distended bladder (Varney, pp. 624-625).

96. **(b)** The white cell count may be elevated to between 15,000 to 20,000 mm^3 the first several days postpartum. A temperature up to 100.4° F may occur in the first 24 hours postpartum as a result of the exertion and dehydration of labor (Ladwig, et al., pp. 711-712).

97. **(d)** For women who choose not to breast feed, suppression of lactation may be enhanced by wearing a supportive, well fitting brassiere continuously for the first 5 to 7 days postpartum, removing the bra only for showering. When showering, she should avoid letting warm water directly hit her breasts as this has a stimulating effect. Warm compresses would also have a stimulating effect. Although bromocriptine was used in the past for lactation suppression, it is no longer recommended due to potential adverse reactions (Ladewig, et al., p. 736).

98. **(a)** Most nonlactating women will resume menses within 4 to 6 weeks of delivery and most women will have ovulated by 45 days after delivery. Contraception should be initiated by the beginning of the fourth postpartum week for the nonlactating woman if she wishes to avoid pregnancy (Hatcher, et al., pp. 591, 598).

99. **(b)** LAM with perfect use is considered to be 98% effective for the first six months in the woman who has not had her first postpartum menses. Perfect use includes nursing on demand (intervals should not exceed four hours during the day and six hours at night), infrequent or no supplementation, and avoidance of the use of pacifiers. It is believed that frequent and strong suckling suppresses ovulation by its effect on GnRH and LH levels (Hatcher, et al., p. 591-594).

100. **(c)** According to the American Academy of Pediatrics' Committee on Nutrition, supplementation of iron is not usually needed before the age of 4 to 6 months. While the iron that is normally found in breast milk may be at lower concentrations than that in prepared formulas, it is better absorbed by the infant. Generally, if mother is well nourished and taking a multivitamin, the only supplement the infant may need in the first six months is fluoride (Ladewig, et al., p. 595).

101. **(d)** Symptoms of subinvolution include a history of prolonged lochia followed by leukorrhea and irregular heavy bleeding. Examination findings include a soft uterus that is larger than normal for the number of weeks postpartum.

If the temperature is elevated or the uterus is tender, endometritis should be suspected (Varney, p. 679).

102. **(a)** Ice has been shown to be the best treatment in the first 24 hour period, but after this time may be detrimental to wound healing. Heat is more effective after the first 24 hours (Varney, p. 646).

103. **(c)** A late postpartum hemorrhage is one that occurs after the first 24 hours following delivery. It occurs most often between 6 to 10 days after delivery and is due to retained placental fragments, infection, or subinvolution. The normal course of postpartum bleeding is lochia rubra (red) which lasts up to three days, lochia serosa (pink) which lasts 3 to 10 days, and lochia alba (yellowish white) which lasts 10 to 21 days (Varney, p. 679).

104. **(d)** Predisposing factors for mastitis include trauma to the breast (cracked nipples), primiparity, lactation, and stasis of breast milk. Actual signs of mastitis include rapid elevation of temperature to 103° to 104° F, increased pulse rate, chills, malaise, headache, and an area on the breast that is red, tender and hard. Treatment includes antibiotic therapy, rest, frequent breast feeding with emptying of the breasts to prevent stasis, and analgesics for pain and fever (Varney, p. 677).

105. **(b)** One of the most common side effects of epidural anesthesia is maternal hypotension with a resultant fetal bradycardia. Trace amounts of anesthetic are absorbed but there is no significant effect on the fetus. Loss of bladder sensation may occur leading to urinary retention. If this does occur, catheterization may be necessary during labor or the immediate postpartum. Although there is controversy regarding the effect on the progress of labor, some studies indicate that the use of epidural anesthesia may slow the progress of labor (ACOG, 1996c, pp. 4-5).

106. **(a)** Postpartum depression usually starts later than postpartum blues and may start anytime during the first year postpartum. Risk factors for postpartum depression include primiparity, ambivalence about the pregnancy, history of postpartum depression or bipolar illness, lack of social support, lack of stable relationship with parents or partner, and dissatisfaction with self. Treatment measures include medication, individual or group psychotherapy, support groups and assistance with childcare and other demands of daily

living. Postpartum psychosis has an incidence of 1 to 2 per 1000 and usually is evident within three months postpartum (Ladewig, et al., p. 788).

107. **(b)** There are three sequential time periods during which attachment and bonding between parents and baby develop and take place. These are the prenatal period, the time of birth and immediately postpartum, and the postpartum and early care taking time (Varney, p. 629).

108. **(c)** In a pudendal block, anesthetic is injected transvaginally into the pudendal nerve which results in numbing of the perineum and outer vaginal area. It is not effective for labor pain but is used to numb the perineal area for delivery and/or repair (Varney, pp. 444-445, 817).

References

American College of Obstetricians and Gynecologists. (1998). *Vaginal birth after previous cesarean delivery.* ACOG Practice Bulletin 2. Washington, DC: ACOG.

American College of Obstetricians and Gynecologists. (1996a). *Assessment of fetal lung maturity.* ACOG Technical Bulletin 230. Washington, DC: ACOG

American College of Obstetricians and Gynecologists. (1996b). *Maternal serum screening.* ACOG Technical Bulletin 228. Washington, DC: ACOG.

American College of Obstetricians and Gynecologists. (1996c). *Obstetric analgesia and anesthesia.* ACOG Technical Bulletin 225. Washington, DC: ACOG.

Carlson, B., & Parrish, D. (1998). Exercising during pregnancy: What to tell your patients. *Women's Health in Primary Care, 1*(2), 171-179.

Centers for Disease Control and Prevention (CDC). (1998). 1998 Guidelines for treatment of sexually transmitted diseases. *MMWR, 47* (No. RR-1), 93-94.

Department of Health and Human Services (DHSS). (1998). *Clinician's handbook of preventive services: Put prevention into practice* (2nd ed.). Washington DC: U.S. Government Printing Office.

Gabbe, S. G., Niebyl, J. R., & Simpson, J. L. (1996). *Obstetrics: Normal and problem pregnancies* (3rd ed.). NY: Churchill Livingstone.

Hatcher, R. A., Trussel, J., Stewart, F., Cates, W., Stewart, G. K., Guest, F., & Kowal, O. (1998). *Contraceptive technology* (17th ed.). New York: Ardent Media.

Hauth, J., & Merenstein, G. (Eds.). (1997) *Guidelines for perinatal care* (4th ed.). Elk Grove, IL: American Academy of Pediatrics and American College of Obstetricians and Gynecologists.

Ladewig, P., London, M., & Olds, S. (1998). *Essentials of maternal-newborn nursing* (4th ed.). Redwood City, CA: Addison-Wesley Nursing.

Niswander, K., & Evans, A. (1996). *Manual of obstetrics* (5th ed.). Boston: Little, Brown & Co.

Pagana, K., & Pagana, T. (1998). *Mosby's manual of diagnostic and laboratory tests.* St. Louis: Mosby.

Varney, H. (1997). *Varney's midwifery* (3rd ed.). Sudbury, MA: Jones & Bartlett Publishers.

Professional Issues

Beth Kelsey

Select one best answer to the following questions.

1. The research method that uses a subjective approach to describe life experiences and give them meaning is:

   a. Correlational
   b. Qualitative
   c. Quasi-experimental
   d. Quantitative

2. A research study is designed to determine if providing information about contraceptive methods to a high school class will reduce the number of pregnancies that occur prior to graduation. The ninth grade class will be provided with information on contraceptive methods, and the tenth grade class will not be given any information. The number of pregnancies that occur prior to graduation in both classes will be compared. The dependent variable in this study is:

   a. Contraceptive information
   b. Number of pregnancies
   c. The ninth grade class
   d. The tenth grade class

3. One measure of central tendency is the median. The median of the following values (9,10,10,12,15,16,18) is:

   a. 10
   b. 12
   c. 14
   d. 15

4. The statement that predicts the expected relationship between two or more variables in a study is the:

    a. Analysis of variance
    b. Level of significance
    c. Hypothesis
    d. Research design

5. You are reading a research study that was designed to measure the occurrence of postpartum depression in adolescent mothers. After reading the study, you question weather the instrument used in the study was actually able to measure postpartum depression in adolescent mothers. What is it about the study that you are questioning?

    a. Reliability
    b. Generalization
    c. Significance
    d. Validity

6. Regulations detailing how Medicare will reimburse for medical services provided by NPs were issued in 1998. Which of the following requirements of the new regulations remains unchanged from previous requirements?

    a. An NP must bill for services as "incident to" a physician's services
    b. A physician must be on site when the services are rendered by the NP
    c. Only an NP working in rural areas may bill directly for services rendered
    d. The NP must have a collaborative agreement with a physician

7. The "reasonable person standard" is used to describe one of the components necessary for:

    a. Breach of duty
    b. Informed consent
    c. Intentional torts
    d. Standards of practice

8. A 28-year-old woman recently had a hysterectomy for invasive cervical cancer. She has filed a malpractice suit against the clinician who performed her Pap smear three years ago. The Pap smear result showed a high grade lesion. Pap smears prior to that were normal. In accordance with the clinic's protocol, three attempts were made to contact the patient. The third attempt was sent by certified mail. This letter came back showing that the patient had moved leaving no forwarding address. Which element, that must be proved by the patient for a malpractice suit based on negligence, is absent?

    a. Duty

    b. Breach of duty

    c. Actual damages

    d. Causation

9. A malpractice claim is made against a nurse practitioner in 1997. The incident related to the claim occurred in 1994. Which of the following types of liability policies would cover this claim?

    a. Claims made coverage policy in 1993 that lapsed in 1996

    b. Claims made policy purchased in 1998 with tail coverage

    c. Occurrence based coverage policy in 1993 that lapsed in 1996

    d. Occurrence based coverage policy that was purchased in 1997

10. Which of the following is not currently regulated by a governmental agency?

    a. Medicare reimbursement

    b. National NP certification

    c. Nurse practice acts

    d. Prescriptive authority

Answers and Rationale

1. **(b)** Qualitative research methods use a systematic, subjective approach to describe life experiences and give them meaning. This type of research is conducted to describe and promote understanding of human experiences such as pain, loss, powerlessness, and caring. Quantitative research uses a formal, objective, and systematic process in which numerical data are utilized to obtain information, describe variables, examine relationships between variables, and determine cause and effect. Correlational and quasi-experimental research are both types of quantitative research (Burns & Grove, p. 791).

2. **(b)** The dependent variable in a study is the response, behavior, or outcome that is predicted or explained in research. Changes in the dependent variable (number of pregnancies) are presumed to be caused by the independent variable (contraceptive information). The ninth grade class is the experimental group and the tenth grade class is the control group (Burns & Grove, p. 779).

3. **(b)** The median is the score or number at the exact center of a group of numbers. Three numbers fall on either side of 12 so it is the median value. Other measures of central tendency include the mean, the mode, and standard deviation (Burns & Grove, p. 786).

4. **(c)** The hypothesis is a formal statement of the expected relationship between two or more variables in a specified population. The hypothesis in the study described in question # 2 might be that providing contraceptive information to high school students in the ninth grade will reduce the number of pregnancies that occur prior to graduation by 50% (Burns & Grove, p. 783).

5. **(d)** A valid instrument measures the construct that it is intended to measure. Reliability is concerned with how consistently an instrument measures the concept of interest. Generalization extends the implications of the findings from the sample studied to the larger population. Significance can either refer to results that are in keeping with those identified by the researcher, or the statistically determined level of significance (Burns & Grove, pp. 783, 792, 795, 798).

6. **(d)** HCFA published final regulations in November 1998 stating that the services of NPs will be eligible for Medicare B coverage and direct payment regardless of the geographic area in which the services are provided. The "incident to" provision is no longer a requirement for reimbursement, nor does a physician have to be on site. A collaborative agreement is still a requirement. HCFA defines collaboration as "a process in which the nurse practitioner has a relationship with one or more physicians to deliver health care services. Such collaboration is to be evidenced by nurse practitioners documenting the nurse practitioner's scope of practice and indicating the relationships that they have with physicians to deal with issues outside their scope of practice. Nurse practitioners must document this process with physicians" (Buppert, pp. 10, 27-28).

7. **(b)** The "reasonable person standard" applies to informed consent. Whether a patient's consent to a procedure was informed depends on whether the health care provider who performed the procedure disclosed all of the facts, risks, and alternatives that a reasonable person would need to make a decision (Urbanski, p. 46).

8. **(b)** Breach of duty means that the clinician failed to perform a duty that she had to the patient. In this situation, the duty is to inform a patient of the abnormal results of a Pap smear. The clinician followed the clinic's protocol and made three attempts to contact the patient, including a certified letter that was returned indicating that the patient had moved and left no forwarding address. This would generally be considered to have met the duty of the clinician. Actual damages would be the hysterectomy and loss of fertility. Not having the Pap smear results may have delayed early treatment that might have been less extensive, preserving the uterus (Dickason, et al., p. 9).

9. **(c)** An occurrence based policy provides coverage for any incident that occurred during the time the policy was in effect. The incident occurred in 1994 so it would be covered by an occurrence based policy that was in effect from 1993 through 1996. Claims made policies cover the individual for any suit filed while the policy is in effect. A claims made policy that lapsed in 1996 would not cover a suit that was filed in 1997. A claims made policy that did not go into effect until 1998 would not cover the suit filed in 1997. Tail coverage extends claims made coverage into the future to cover claims filed after the basic claims coverage period (Hawkins & Thibodeau, p. 102; Moskosky, p. 478).

10. **(b)** National NP certification is provided by a variety of nongovernmental agencies including the American Nurses Credentialing Center (ANCC), the National Certification Corporation (NCC), and the National Association of Pediatric Nurse Associates and Practitioners (NAPNAP). Medicare reimbursement is under the jurisdiction of the Health Care Financing Administration (HCFA). Nurse Practice Acts are defined by individual State nursing boards. Prescriptive authority involves State nursing boards and in some States also involves medical and pharmacy boards (Hawkins & Thibodeau, pp. 82, 86, 93-97).

References

Burns, N., & Grove, S. (1997). *The practice of nursing research: Conduct, critique, and utilization* (3rd ed.). Philadelphia: W. B. Saunders.

Buppert, C. (1998). HCFA releases final rules on PA and NP medicare reimbursement. *Clinician News*, 2(6), 1, 10, 27-28.

Dickason, E., Silverman, B., & Kaplan, J. (1998). *Maternal-infant nursing care* (3rd ed.). St. Louis: Mosby.

Hawkins, J., & Thibodeau, J. (1996). *The advanced practice nurse: Current issues* (4th ed.). New York: The Tiresias Press.

Moskosky, S. (Ed.). (1995). *Women's health care nurse practitioner certification review guide*. Potomac, MD: Health Leadership Associates, Inc.

Urbanski, P. (1997). Getting the go ahead: Helping patients understand informed consent. *AWHONN Lifelines*, June, 45-48.

Wysocki, S. (1997). Medicare reimbursement for NPs passes into law—what does it mean to your practice? *Reprocussions*, Winter, 1-3.

Health Leadership Associates
Nurse Practitioner Continuing Education
Programs

Analysis of the 12-lead ECG

This course is designed for advanced practice nurses. During this 8 hour course you will review cardiac electrophysiology, the cardiac cycle and cardiac muscle function as a basis for 12-lead ECG interpretation; analysis of dysrhythmia, conduction abnormalities, atrial abnormalities, ventricular hypertrophy, axis deviation, myocardial ischemia and myocardial infarction. A one hour practice workshop completes the program. A comprehensive course syllabus is included.

Pharmacology for Nurse Practitioners: A Comprehensive
Review and Update

This 30 hour course is designed as a comprehensive presentation and review of pharmacology from the physiologic perspective. In addition to presenting the pharmacokinetics and pharmacodynamics of drugs (indications, contraindications, mechanisms of action, excretion and side effects profile) the corresponding body system physiology will be presented in a format that makes the pharmacology easy to understand and apply in clinical practice. A comprehensive course syllabus is included.

Suturing Review and Practice

This $2\frac{1}{2}$ hour course is designed for nurse practitioners who do not have significant suturing experience. Whether you have been taught but haven't practiced, or have never been taught at all, this program will introduce and reinforce skills that you have not had the opportunity to develop. A brief didactic session on wound assessment and preparation is followed by hands-on instruction and practice of the simple interrupted and vertical mattress techniques.

For information on these and other programs contact:
Health Leadership Associates, Inc.
P.O. Box 59153
Potomac, MD 20859
1-800-435-4775

For information on Certification Review Courses, Home Study Programs and Review Books contact:

Health Leadership Associates, Inc.
Post Office Box 59153
Potomac, Maryland 20859

1-800-435-4775

NOTES

NOTES

NOTES

NOTES